Nurses
Beyond
Borders

Nurses
Beyond
Borders

True Stories
of Heroism and
Healing Around the World

Nancy Leigh Harless, ARNP
Editor

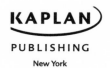

KAPLAN

PUBLISHING

New York

© 2010 Kaplan, Inc.

Published by Kaplan Publishing, a division of Kaplan, Inc.
1 Liberty Plaza, 24th Floor
New York, NY 10006

The stories in this anthology are based on real events; however, names, places, and other details have been changed for the sake of privacy.

ISBN-13: 978-1-60978-204-7

Contents

PART TWO: IN THE SHADOWS

PART THREE: FINDING HUMOR

PART FOUR: LOOKING BACK

Introduction

As the traveler who has once been from home is wiser than he who has never left his own doorstep, so a knowledge of one other culture should sharpen our ability to scrutinize more steadily, to appreciate more lovingly, our own.

~ Margaret Mead

TRAVEL AND WORKING abroad has a way of stretching us. As our awareness of a wider world and other traditions expands, so does our capacity for compassion and love. This is the message, written between the lines, and repeated over and over in the stories of *Nurses Beyond Borders*. I am in awe of each of the nurses who have shared their personal, heartfelt stories. Each touched many lives, and in that doing was in turn deeply changed.

There can be no one description that fits these special people. Their nursing roles were many, as were their reasons for traveling. Some went as teachers to train the next generation of nurses. Some went to improve the quality of a people's lives by providing healthcare in a foreign clinic or hospital; some opened new clinics in villages where before there had been no healthcare. They *all* went with the intention, on some level, to save lives and alleviate suffering.

As nurses, when we experience working in a new and different environment—perhaps with fewer resources than what we are accustomed to—we learn "up close and personal" how others live and how they provide healthcare, however meager it may be. We adapt our practices to fit within both the culture and the resources available to us. Our nursing framework of ideal practices is ejected, replaced with the need to do what we can, with what we have. In the story "Susy," we witness an emergency cesarean section in an 8-by-10-foot concrete room full of rainwater; in "The Lucky Ones," we frantically search the tiny hospital with nurse Tess for a portable oxygen tank, but none is found. In "The Gift of David," a premature baby boy lies for three days in the incubator, a gift from a very kind donor. The problem is that there is no power to run it. All of the nurses of *Nurses Beyond Borders* demonstrate flexibility and creativity in their international nursing practices. They make do with what they have.

Each has a deep respect for the people they worked with and for their customs. In "Waterlife," John Fiddler finds creative ways around local customs while at the same time being respectful of the culture's mores. Nurse researcher Julia Quiring-Emblen reverently discusses the differences and similarities between Native American healers and typical western nursing practices in her story "Frog Leaves, Sage, and Cedar." The nurses' cultural awareness and respect also extends to the healthcare professionals in the country where they work. Maribeth Diver clearly states this concept in her story, "A Midwife in Laos": "Every single healthcare provider—especially the midwife—holds fast to deep-rooted clinical beliefs and practices. And this is no less true for practitioners in underprivileged countries." All of the nurses who shared their stories for this anthology understand this basic tenet and express high admiration for the local healthcare providers with whom they worked.

Some of the stories speak of the importance in learning the local language; others emphasize that communication is universal, not only with language but also through gestures and laughter. All agree that the principles of patience, tolerance, compassion, and cultural sensitivity speak volumes in any language.

Some of the nurse contributors to *Nurses Beyond Borders* stood very close to the edge and bore witness to violence, atrocities, and neglect in the course of their work. In "The Small Scheme of Life," Mary Catlin looks back at the horror, and the madness, of working in a refugee camp in Rwanda— "a very tilted place." In "Breath," Joan Cantwell reflects on a woman who walked 100 land mine–laced miles to come to a Thailand hospital. In "Journey to the Mekong Delta," Cheri Clark whisks ten babies, many sick and in need of immediate medical attention, out of a country in the grips of one of the deadliest wars in modern history.

But certainly not all of the stories are from areas of war or unrest, nor are they necessarily all stories from poverty-ridden countries. Many of the stories tell of the joyful lives of those who have very little in the way of material things—of the simplicity that defines their life. Over time the nurses learn that relationships to nature—and relationships between people—become the priority when things are spare. And they return home humbled, more aware of the plenty, and of the waste, in their homeland.

The amazing nurses of *Nurses Beyond Borders* travel abroad to work, or work in their home country, with people very different from themselves. They are undeniably very special people who reach out eagerly—though not necessarily without fear—for new, rich experiences. They provide care and compassion to all those in need. These extraordinary nurses lead wide lives. Once they experience transcultural nursing they are forever changed; their view of the world broadens; their sense of self deepens. They know in their bones they are a part of the web of life on a global scale. In the words of contributor Tess Deshefy-Longhi, in her story by the same name, these nurses are indeed "The Lucky Ones."

Sit back. Get comfortable. Be carried away to China, Honduras, South Africa, Cambodia, Finland, Swaziland, and beyond. And then get uncomfortable—*very* uncomfortable—so uneasy that you, too, feel the call to action. There is much work to be done. My personal hope is that this amazing collection of nurses' stories about practicing both the art and the science of their profession will ignite a spark in others to reach out to the larger world. I hope this book inspires...*you.*

Nurses
Beyond
Borders

PART ONE

Times of Transition

Mae Mae

~

Elizabeth Coulter, RN

The old man found the bundle in a pile of rags under the bench on his way home from the factory. He might not have noticed the whimper had the heat not caused him to sit and rest. When he unwrapped the curious bundle he expected to find a cat or perhaps a small dog, but to his surprise, it was a baby! Not only was it a girl—which was already a disadvantage—but her face was disfigured. Her upper lip was split in two places, leaving an opening from her mouth into her nose. Many of the townsfolk were stuck in the old ways. Fear and superstition must have caused the mother to leave the helpless infant beside the bench to die or to be found by a benevolent person. The old man picked the baby up in his arms and continued down the road to his house. He hoped his wife would understand.

WHEN CINDY ASKED whether I wanted to join her on a medical mission to China, I said yes, partly because I loved to travel and partly because I didn't think she'd follow through. We worked in a busy emergency room in Seattle and were always looking for opportunities that would whet our appetite for the profession. After many years of ER nursing, my enthusiasm for helping people had atrophied and my empathy was as pliable as rigor mortis. To my surprise, Cindy contacted the organization Love Without Boundaries, and before I knew it, we were on our way to Luoyang, China, as a part of a Surgical Cleft Palate/Lip Team.

"Kids are simple," I reassured Cindy as we settled in our hotel room after the long flight. She and I would be responsible for running the recovery/pediatric ward. "Maintain their airway and they'll breathe."

I personally knew how important a patent airway was in a child. My son had a seizure disorder, which started when he was only three months old. He was "status"— that is, his seizures wouldn't stop without intravenous medication—so we were regulars in our local emergency room. My experience with him influenced my decision to return to school when he was ten, to study nursing. Unfortunately, a year after my graduation, he had a seizure that landed him in the ER. After the sedating drugs stopped the seizure, I left the room to send my husband home to watch our other children. When I returned, my son had stopped breathing and a nurse was doing CPR.

Without rule number one, airway, you don't get rule number two, breathing. He died when he was 11 years old.

After turning out the light, I said good night to Cindy and tried to sleep. As usual, in the stillness of the night my mind began to race. I wondered how healthy the babies would be and what kind of resuscitation equipment would be available. I tossed and turned. It wasn't the hard mattress that kept me awake, nor the sound of Cindy's snoring, but the awareness that I had never seen a baby with an unrepaired cleft lip or palate and had no idea what to expect.

There were 30 members of our team, including two surgeons and anesthesiologists and ten nurses; the rest were nonmedical volunteers. The volunteers were versatile people who did everything from interviewing potential patients to making sure the team was fed. They ran errands and kept all of us happy.

After a fitful night, I stared through the window on the bus and watched the early morning on the sidewalks of Luoyang. There were multiple layers of life—a veritable "Where's Waldo" of activity—on our way to the orphanage where we would be working. Team One had arrived the previous week and set up a temporary two-room operating suite and recovery room on the top floor of the orphanage. The director had graciously allowed us to take over the entire top floor, but requested that we respect the privacy of the orphans who lived there. We were not allowed to enter the large double doors into the orphanage proper.

As we pulled through the gates, little faces peered through grime-covered windows. We must have been a distraction for the curious children, who were quickly shooed away by an unseen adult. I picked up a bag of equipment and walked up the wide steps of the staircase. A montage of handprints waist-high on the wall of the stairway and the sound of voices reciting in unison on one floor, and then singing on another, were evidence of the children of all ages who called the orphanage home.

The eighth floor housed the operating rooms, recovery room, and a large room that served as our pediatric ward, which was already filled with rows of alternating cots and cribs, and parents and children. The melodic sounds of Mandarin echoed over crying children. Anxious parents held children tightly in their arms while they waited for surgery, while post-op parents smiled, waiting for discharge. The two night nurses from Team One gave Cindy and me report at the nurses' station, a folding table and a shelf that held supplies.

As we planned our day, a little boy broke free from his father and ran over to us. His smile wasn't stunted by his cleft lip. I bent down and let him pat my curly, red hair. He gently pulled a single curl, laughed as it bounced back, then ran back to his cot to wait for surgery in the arms of his father.

Fortunately, our background in the ER meant Cindy and I were used to bringing order from chaos, and the noise level didn't bother us. We separated the fresh post-op children from those preparing for discharge. Parents talked excitedly and joined in as we slid their cots and cribs to the right side of the room. Gestures and smiles replaced words until our interpreter showed up.

As children were discharged, groggy ones fresh from surgery appeared. The ages of our patients varied from eight months to ten years. Orphanage nannies left the drowsy patients to sleep, while parents were fearful of picking up their children and disturbing the children's much-needed rest. I had already been warned by the lead surgeon that the Chinese had a tendency to lay babies down on their backs for hour and hours, sometimes all day, resulting in flat heads. I doubted my brief instruction would sway tradition, but I assured the doctor I would try.

As the pace turned frantic, it was difficult keeping patients straight. With no room numbers or ID bands, and our inability to speak the language, monitoring individual oral intake and frequent vital signs proved frustrating and nearly impossible. Cindy came up with the brilliant idea of hourly rounds. At the top of each hour, we marched between rows of cribs, blowing bubbles into the air, singing songs while taking temperatures and stamping happy faces on chubby hands. We instructed caregivers to pick up and jostle their children, stimulating them to cry. The parents looked at us as if we were crazy, so Daniel, our Chinese translator, explained our rationale. Crying would force oxygen deep into their lungs.

When my son was alive, I believed everything in life brought meaning. Believing that no experience was random helped me through every difficult hurdle that came along. In our makeshift hospital, holding a baby with a freshly sutured upper lip in my arms, I wondered if luck, and luck only, determined your path. Most likely, my son wouldn't have lived past a year in Luoyang.

Mae Mae had a dream that someday she would meet some good-hearted people. She never told anyone, because she had learned not to expect miracles. They appeared only in storybooks.

Years ago she learned about the surgery that would repair the deformity on her upper lip. She knew that if her family had more money, she could look like other girls. But her father was an old man and still worked long hours in the chemical factory, pulling coal residues from the furnace. How could she complain, when he never did, even though his shoulder hunched forward and his back ached?

Although he could not read, her father believed that education would free his children from the impoverished life they inherited. As a result, Mae Mae studied harder than her brother and sister and scored in the top of her class. At school, ignorant girls looked at her with cold eyes and made cruel, snobbish comments, so she sat alone and hid her deformity behind a book. At 16 years old, she wanted to dream like other girls. She never told anyone, but she was lonely.

Last night, a neighbor came to their house and told her father about the foreigners who had come to Luoyang to do surgery for free. Her father looked at

Mae Mae and promised he would do everything in his power to take her to Luoyang.

On the third day, I was asked to go to the second floor to give antibiotics to two babies who'd had surgery the previous week and were reportedly not doing well. A nanny led us down a poorly lit hall, passing room after room filled with small cribs. The side rails of the cribs were lower than those of standard cribs in America—a baby could easily flip over. But these babies lay docilely on their backs. I recalled what the surgeon had said about the flat heads of orphans.

The first patient was an 11-month-old who had developed a fever. She was tiny, about the size of a four-month-old American baby. Her lip incision was healing well, but her breathing was rapid and shallow. I picked her warm body up and jostled her. She immediately cried—a reassuring sign. I instructed Daniel to tell the nanny that the baby needed to drink every two hours. She smiled and nodded, but with so many babies under her care, the chance of my request being carried out was slim.

The other baby, a tiny eight-month-old, looked sicker. She barely cried when I stimulated her. I treated her fever with Tylenol and persevered until she drank a full bottle of water. With the hydration, her floppy arms stiffened and grabbed at the bottle. The nanny assured me she would watch both babies closely.

As we walked past rows upon rows of cribs, I wondered how the two small babies would fare. Daniel and

I walked up the back stairs and peeked into the gymnasiums, where children played and studied. On one floor, a girl pushed a wheelchair that held a little child with cerebral palsy. On another, children sat reciting lessons. The children appeared happy and clean, but the rooms were sparely furnished. I asked Daniel what happened to the toys our team had donated. A nanny said they were locked away so the children wouldn't break them.

I then understood the words the surgeon had said at our first meeting. "You can only do what you do."

It was Mae Mae's first trip out of Feng Qiu. The world outside was much more flourishing than she had thought. She walked with her father, side by side, along the road for hours, until a kind man picked them up. After hearing her story, he drove them to the train station and gave them money. She smiled as the country flew past. Every road, every building, and every person was a new opportunity.

There was a buzz among the operating room nurses when Cindy and I arrived the next morning. A father and his 16-year-old daughter, who had a bilateral lip, had arrived outside the orphanage gates during the night. They had waited there until the surgeons arrived. Thankfully, the staff was flexible enough to fit the girl in. Her surgery would be the last of the day.

The day progressed rapidly. Cindy and I had the room running like clockwork and had added dancing as part of our hourly rounds. So far, all our children had recovered well, and even the two babies on the second floor looked better.

Mae Mae lay on the cot and, still drowsy, touched her lip. Her fingers traveled along the stitches, so I took her hand in mine and laid it by her side. She smiled, closed her eyes, and returned to sleep. What once was a gaping hole was a tenderly sutured lip.

Her father wouldn't stop smiling and bowing. He was a thin man, muscles taut from years of hard physical labor. His face wizened with wrinkles, and with a thin, white Fu Manchu mustache, he was the quintessential man of China past. He still wore the traditional Mao uniform, a blue tunic. When the surgeon appeared at his daughter's bedside, her father lay prostrate on the floor. The surgeon crouched down, placed his hand on the father's shoulder, and guided him up. The two men—a skilled surgeon from the United States who had traveled the world helping children, and an old man in a Mao uniform who had given an abandoned baby girl a home—honored each other in true humility.

Mae Mae recovered in a small, private room. She spent most of her time hunched over a journal, writing beautifully scripted Chinese characters on its pages. She was dressed in a new outfit, a gift from some of the nurses. The organization, so impressed with Mae Mae's character and scholastic achievements, had committed to paying for her university tuition.

Daniel translated the thank-you letter that Mae Mae wrote:

My fate has been rewritten. Now I firmly believe in my goal and the way I should go about in my life. In the old time, I was lonely. Now people will look at me and I will be like every other girl. The foreigners are so kind to me. You have given me clothing and will pay my college fees, which is unbelievable and unexpected. I have nothing to give in return. But what I will give is the kindness you have shown to me, I will show to others.

Let's fly freely in our own blue sky, release our dreams and never regret our lives. Be strong no matter how hard it is.

I don't know if our lives are predestined—written in stone and permanently sealed—or if our path is like a feather gently floating downward until a gust of wind blows in another direction. But I do know that my responsibility is to make the best choices possible, to accept the consequences, and to believe in something better, not only for myself but for those around me as well.

Through the window of the bus, I watched an old man walk briskly on the sidewalk. He held a small wooden birdcage, like a lantern, in front of him. Inside, a small black bird flapped its wings. I imagined the song it sang was beautiful.

Carmelita's Hands

~

Martha N. Ezell, MSN, RN

Her name is Carmelita. When we first met, she was a 15-year-old living in a tiny Honduran village called El Vino. I was a member of a medical missions team from the United States visiting her country for a week in March 2003. As we left our bus and climbed the dusty road into the village, it was evident that our visit had been publicized and anticipated. An orderly crowd of about 200 was assembled, patiently waiting outside the only building in sight.

The structure was a plain, industrial-looking building made of cement block walls on a concrete floor. The entire building, inside and out, was painted white and trimmed with an interesting variation of green I'd never seen before. This simple structure would be home to farm equipment or ski boats in our privileged homeland, but here in Honduras the humble building proudly served as El Vino's city hall, school, market, and church. On this day, the building would temporarily become a grocery, department store, clinic, and pharmacy. And for a teenager named Carmelita, it would be the site of a life-changing miracle.

Our group of 30 *gringos* quickly unloaded the bus and truck, and found adequate places in the building to set up the areas of service we planned to provide. The first room was devoted to food distribution, while the second would house the clothing giveaway. The third and fourth rooms became rudimentary dental and medical clinics. The last room, because it housed two sets of rickety, empty bookcases, became the pharmacy.

Word spread quickly and the villagers queued up outside each of the rooms, according to their needs. Children from our group dissolved into the crowd with the assignment of entertaining the Honduran children while parents waited. As is usually the case in Honduras, a soccer game began.

My assignment for the day was to assist one of the dentists. We unwrapped the pieces of equipment the dentist had brought, dipped them in an antiseptic solution, and placed them on a tray atop a wooden table. We set a folding metal chair by the only window and declared ourselves open for business. Our first patient entered the room, holding a piece of paper with two numbers written on it. On the porch outside, a Spanish-speaking dentist had performed a speedy triage, determined the work to be done, and written the information on a scrap of paper. For this patient, two molars would be pulled. Dentistry in countries like Honduras consists mainly of removing the most rotten teeth before infection reaches the bone. Few of the villagers own a toothbrush or know anything about dental hygiene. By middle age, many Hondurans are toothless.

The dentist conducted an examination of our patient's mouth, identified the two decayed molars, injected the patient with lidocaine, and went to work. My job was to hold a flashlight in one hand and the tray of instruments in the other. Patient after patient, hour after hour, the work continued. Countless teeth were extracted, bleeding was compressed, sutures were sewn, and *Dios te bendiga's* (God bless you's) were exchanged. As each patient left, he or she was directed to a group of American teenagers to be presented with the gift of a toothbrush, a tube of toothpaste, and a cheery brushing demonstration.

In the early afternoon, Carmelita was directed to our chair. She handed me the piece of paper containing her dental diagnosis and silently sat down. She sat as many nervous people do, with hands tucked under legs and feet tucked under the chair. Despite her youth and beauty, her face seemed frozen in fear. She refused to look at me or hold my hands as I knelt beside her to introduce myself. She wore an oddly mismatched outfit and dime-store flip-flops on her dusty feet.

As the dentist began to work, Carmelita's fear became tangible. I put down the tray of instruments, put my hands on her shaking knees, and attempted to offer comfort. Fear overcame hesitancy and she frantically squeezed my hands. Then I saw them. From each of her lovely, caramel-colored hands stretched not five, but six fingers. My mind struggled to process what I was seeing. Polydactyly, I thought, remembering the word and picture in my medical dictionary. I realized that what I'd interpreted as shyness or fear was more accurately shame. Carmelita didn't want to hold my hands. Doing so would risk exposing her own, and the shame of her deformity. I quietly called to my mother, who was working nearby, and asked her to go get the doctor.

Moments later I heard the booming voice of a friend and team member, a renowned head and neck cancer surgeon from Vanderbilt University Medical Center in Nashville, Tennessee. He is the kind of skilled physician people wait six months to see. Carmelita waited two minutes. Without alerting Carmelita, who thankfully had her head back and mouth open, the doctor examined her hands as I held them. After a quick assessment, he told me in English that although the extra digits looked like functioning fingers, they actually contained no bones and could easily be removed.

When Carmelita's dental work was completed, Emily, our translator, was called into service. "Carmelita," she said in perfect Spanish, "this is our doctor. He sees that you have some extra fingers. He knows how to remove them. Would you like for him to do this?"

Her face twisted in disbelief. She looked from Emily

to me to the physician, seeking verification of the amazing message. Then, despite the huge wads of gauze in her mouth, Carmelita broke into a huge smile and said, "*Si, si, si!*" At this point, Carmelita pointed to her dusty feet. We saw twelve toes.

Three wooden school desks were placed end-to-end to be used as the operating table. Surgical instruments and sterile drapes appeared. A medical student from Oklahoma and I would assist the physician, while other members of our team were recruited to entertain and comfort Carmelita. One volunteer stood nearby with a piece of cardboard he used to gently fan away flies from the surgical area. Earphones attached to a portable CD player were presented to our patient, in hopes that the novelty of the device as well as the calming music would offer a diversion. Carmelita's hands and feet were scrubbed with soap and water, then antiseptic wash, and finally Betadine. The scene was surreal to me. No consent forms were signed. There were no consults, no pre-op blood work, no fasting, no anesthesia, and certainly no insurance approvals. I am, however, fairly certain a few prayers were offered as the procedure began.

In less than an hour, Carmelita's four amputated digits lay in a bowl. Her wounds were carefully sutured and bandaged. Prescription antibiotics and analgesics came from the pharmacy next door. With the help of our translator, the physician gave postoperative instructions to Carmelita. Curious and happy friends came to escort her home.

We were told later that while polydactyly is not particularly uncommon in Honduras, it is considered an embarrassing and shameful condition. It is impossible to understand the lifetime of humiliation caused by Carmelita's extra fingers and toes. It was easy to see her joy at being freed from them. I was reminded that all healthy humans feel the desire to fit in, to be regarded as "normal." For Carmelita, an American doctor had, in an hour, removed the deformity that had defined the entirety of her young life.

One year later, our group returned to El Vino. The first person we saw running from the village to meet us was Carmelita. She was not alone. She had brought two relatives to meet the physician, pointing to their extra fingers and toes. More miracles would occur that day.

As American healthcare professionals, we often take our blessings for granted. We work with a staff surrounded by skilled, well-educated professionals. We practice in comfortable, modern hospitals that are warm in the winter and cool in the summer. We have at our disposal the latest diagnostic technology and tools. We are comfortable. My encouragement to all who read this is to get uncomfortable, if even for one week. Seek an opportunity to go somewhere like Honduras. Go and take your children. Share your skill and compassion with someone like Carmelita. The life you change may be your own.

My life is changed each time I venture beyond the borders of my safe and familiar homeland. I fall in love with the sweet smiles and happy voices of Honduran children. I long for the simplicity that defines their life! I admire the sacrifices of the mothers who give all they have to keep their children safe and healthy. I grieve for those who can't be helped or healed. I miss them when I leave. And each time I come home, for just a little while I remember how blessed I am and how privileged to share those blessings with my friends—my *amigos* in Honduras.

Frog Leaves, Sage, and Cedar

~

Julia Quiring-Emblen, PhD, RN

As PART OF a grounded theory research study, a colleague and I interviewed a number of First Nations people (the term used for Native Americans residing in British Columbia, Canada) to learn about the spiritual aspects of their health beliefs and practices. Upon inquiry in and around the reservation, I was referred to Bea (not her real name) because she was known as a local healer. Meeting her over lunch, I was most impressed with Bea and the lifetime of healing practices she quietly recounted to me.

Bea grew up in the Fraser Valley of the lower British Columbia mainland. She was one of the Sto:lo Coast Salish natives indigenous to this area. She told me that natives often took the name of land owners in the area or other Europeans living nearby. Bea told me that Sto:lo means "river" and is used to refer to natives living along the Fraser River and its tributaries.

As a child, Bea watched other family members pick healing herbs and use them to help people. Unfortunately, they had no herbs strong enough to treat her tuberculosis, so she spent a number of her teen years in a sanatorium being cared for by Catholic Sisters. Because of this experience she incorporated many Catholic spiritual practices into her healing approaches, using them along with her knowledge of native practices and beliefs regarding healing.

Bea described many of the approaches she used for healing both in her work in a native clinic and in her own personal healing practice. She shared details and stories about using various herbs, longhouse experiences, and other general beliefs.

Bea used the knowledge she gained as a child from her maternal grandparents to choose different herbs for healing. She gathered a lot of herbs, including something she called "frog legs," as well as plantain, and made teas or poultices with these for the patient to drink or apply. She chose each herb for its specific healing properties related to infections, coughs, bleeding, and a host of other conditions.

Bea told me about using sage in "smudging." Occasionally she was asked to help college students who were having trouble with their university studies. She would bring a group together in a circle, put a smudge pot in the middle with some sage, and burn it. While the scent of sage wafted through the room air, the students were encouraged to talk. She provided an eagle's feather to pass around, with the rule that only the person holding the feather could speak. In Sto:lo culture the eagle is a symbol of wisdom, as it flies overhead and sees all things. Using the feather prevented several students from speaking at once. When conversation about feelings decreased, Bea added a little more sage to the pot so that more people could speak and release their negative feelings.

Cedar is considered a cleansing agent. Many homes place cedar over their doors so that when people enter the home, their thoughts and stresses are released and they can bring a free, relaxed mind into the house. Bea also used cedar to brush people, starting at the head and brushing down to the feet to rid the person of stresses and other negative aspects.

Bea described longhouses as being places people entered when it grew cold and where they remained until the spring thaw. She said that longhouses often were used to treat those who had alcohol or drug problems. A fire was kept burning (until the toxic effects of smoke were recognized; eventually the fire was replaced with a gas stove). The Elders—senior members of a tribal group— were the ones to make such logistical decisions, as well as to provide social and spiritual counsel.

In the longhouses, people took turns cooking so that all could participate in the songs and spirit-dances. Bea told me that for years she had danced in the evenings, but somehow never received her "song." One day while dancing she suddenly received her song. This seemed to be a highlight for her in spiritual development.

I asked Bea whether I might bring to her a group of my nursing students who were studying native health beliefs so that she could talk to them about her healing practices. She agreed, and had us meet near a small park. Because it was fall there were few plants growing for herbs, so Bea took the students to a cedar tree and had them break off a small branch. She encouraged them to thank the tree for the branch, which was to be used for health. Bea then showed the students how to brush someone off with a cedar bough to cleanse the person's thoughts and body.

She also took the students to a little stream and showed them how to cup their hands and get a little water. Bea had them put some water on their foreheads and necks as another way of cleansing their bodies.

Bea then described the personal song she had received as a special gift from the Creator. She hummed a few bars of "Amazing Grace," which surprised the students, and she explained that her song was a little like that.

At another time, I asked Bea about some of the special practices identified by others whom I had interviewed. She said that using masks at weddings was a special way to invoke the powers of the animals the masks represented. She told me that some people left food out at anniversaries of the deaths of loved ones and that the next morning the food was gone. The people believe that the loved ones needed it to help sustain them on their journey.

Bea was not particularly focused on the practice of burying a baby's placenta under a tree so the baby would grow strong like the tree, as some other healers had told me. She said that at funerals relatives are not allowed to help cook food for the celebrative feast, because their sadness might enter the food and make the guests ill. Children are not allowed to go to funerals, to prevent the sickness of the spirit of the deceased moving into or taking over the immature spirit of a child.

As Bea and I met over several years, she shared more of the deeper levels of healing experiences. She described an instance when a baby was very ill and did not seem to get better. The healer was able to see a blue light in the baby's esophagus, and he thought this accounted for the baby being unable to keep milk down. The healer could not determine the cause of the illness until he asked the mother if she had gone to the home of an older person during her pregnancy. Immediately prior to her delivery, the mother had visited a relative who was very ill, and after her visit the relative improved.

The healer told the woman that the sick spirit in the relative had transferred to her baby's esophagus, so he prayed that the sick spirit would return to the old man. When the healer saw that the blue light was gone, the baby was able to keep milk down and his health improved. A short time after this, upon the return of his sick spirit, the old man died.

Bea talked about prayers, but she never gave me any clear details about what would be prayed for or how the prayers were made. She did indicate that prayers were made to the spirits and the Great Spirit. I wondered whether this was a point where she had merged her native and Roman Catholic spiritual beliefs.

I did not have contact with Bea for more than a year, and on returning to the community I was told that she had died. Apparently she had fainted in a longhouse ceremony and, though taken to the nearest hospital, did not recover. She had told me of her long-standing kidney disease, and so I surmised that the stress of some of the activities had caused her to faint. I was sorry that Bea had lost consciousness and was unable to use some of her own healing remedies.

Through Bea and other Sto:lo natives whom I interviewed, I had a window into traditional First Nations healing beliefs and practices. Apparently there are many levels of healing in Bea's culture. She had not reached the level of the highest healer, even though she continued taking classes in native and Western medical practices.

I found Bea's approaches quite distinct from my own traditional experience in caring for others using Western medicine. But there are amazing similarities. Like practitioners of Western medicine, Bea initially did a careful assessment—both verbal and physical. She used fewer diagnostic tests than are common in my healthcare. Bea gave people herbs to drink and to apply externally. This is similar to many herbal treatments common in alternative therapies and other pharmacological treatment. She used substances to allow people to become less inhibited in sharing. Similarly, emotional reflection or catharsis is a common psychiatric nursing communication approach.

Longhouse treatment that removes those with abuse problems from general society for a period of time is somewhat like Western medicine's rehabilitation centers for persons to recover from substance abuse using strong support from well-trained personnel. Bea did not use surgical procedures; instead, she used discerning prayer and incantations. In Western medicine prayers may be offered, though not always verbally.

I am indebted to Bea for sharing with me parts of her life as a practicing native healer. My life is enriched because I had the privilege of becoming acquainted with Bea and others, initially for research purposes and then to become friends with Bea. My friendship with her has enriched my understanding of the health beliefs and practices of healers caring for traditional Sto:lo natives. In addition, I learned to know a very special person. Even though she lived with chronic physical illness, she was able to grow and develop herself as a warm, sensitive, and gracious human being.

Some of the cultural beliefs discussed in this story were obtained while conducting interviews with Evelyn Labun, research collaborator, for a grounded theory study on the meaning of health for the Sto:lo.

Ice Cream Days

~

Tilda Shalof, RN, BScN, CNCC(C)

O<small>N MY OWN</small>, high in the sky, enveloped by the gentle roar of the airplane's engines, I was calm. I had no idea where I was going, where I'd stay or find work, but I was thrilled at the prospect of my adventure. Yes, I was finally a Real Nurse and now had the documents to prove it. However, even with my university degree there were few jobs for nurses in Canada. It was the downward swing of the boom-bust economic cycle, and as hospitals downsized, nurses were the first to be cut. I wasn't worried, though, because I had long ago decided on my postgraduation plans: I would go to Israel. I told everyone that I wanted to connect with my Jewish identity. This was true enough, but I kept quiet about my other reasons: I was seeking fun, romance, and danger!

ARRIVING IN ISRAEL, I felt an immediate sense of belonging to the country and its history, even though I knew no one and barely spoke the language. From the airport, I took a bus to the nearest hospital, Tel HaShomer, a large medical center just outside Tel Aviv.

At the hospital, I met the director of nursing, Shoshana Zamir, a tall, commanding woman in a white uniform and sandals. She welcomed me warmly, as though I was her long-lost daughter, and praised my halting Hebrew. It was as if by clasping me to her huge bosom she was enfolding me into the entire country, its history and collective destiny. Yes, indeed, they needed nurses badly, she lamented, especially well-educated ones like me.

Shoshana suggested I start in a general medicine ward where most of the patients were elderly, bedridden, and had chronic illnesses with no cure. She introduced me to Yaffa, the head nurse, who had a roly-poly body, solid as a truck, encased in a crisp white uniform. Sticking straight up on her head was a white winged cap, its corner points sharp as daggers. "Teelda," she said. "What kind of name is zat?" Yaffa made my name sound too much like the word *gleeda*, which was Hebrew for ice cream. She looked me over. "Where's your *kep*?"

"I don't have one," I answered with a superior smile. "Nurses don't wear caps anymore. They're old-fashioned."

"You're not a nurse without zee kep. Wear it tomorrow if you want to work here," Yaffa said.

Well, we'll see about that, I thought.

"Vhat? Again vit no kep?" Yaffa said as soon as she

saw me the next morning. "You are forbidden to take care of patients without zee kep." Yaffa folded her arms across her chest. I stood equally firm. She handed me a mop and a pail. "Here," she said, "Do *sponja*."

I lasted two weeks, hating every minute of it. Every morning I did "*sponja*." It involved filling a bucket of warm soapy water, dumping it out all over the floor, and then sweeping the water outside into the cow pasture behind the hut. Afterward, I folded laundry and gave out lunch trays to patients. It was demoralizing. This wasn't nursing! Luckily, Shoshana came for a visit and saw how miserable I was. I guess she didn't want to lose me, as she offered me a position in a new unit.

"It will be a bone-marrow transplant unit. You will start working in the hematology clinic and when the transplant unit is opened, you'll work there." Hematology involved blood diseases and that meant mostly cancers, such as leukemia and lymphoma. It was an honor to be chosen for the challenge; Shoshana must have seen potential in me.

THE HEMATOLOGY OUTPATIENT CLINIC was a casual place, despite the seriousness of the patients' illnesses. The doctors and nurses all wore loose green scrubs and sandals, and everyone called each other by their first names. Every patient had to have blood tests before seeing the doctor. Aviva Shofet was one of the senior nurses in the clinic. She taught me how to draw blood and start IVs, and soon I got pretty good at it. It was a thrill to see the tiny speck of blood, called the "flashback," in the plastic sheath of the angiocath. It was the surest sign I was in the vein. I discovered that the best way to locate a difficult vein was by touch, and sometimes I even closed my eyes to feel for it. I learned the secret idiosyncratic places in patients' arms and hands where the best veins were hidden. First I got to know a patient's veins, and then I got to know the patient.

After they had their blood drawn, the patients waited to see the doctor, who would examine them and review the results of their tests. Meanwhile, the nurses began the treatments, which usually involved chemotherapy, antibiotics, and/or blood transfusions. An astonishing array of patients came to us in that tiny clinic.

A bedouin shepherd arrived for his chemotherapy, directly from tending his sheep. He had dark skin and a bushy white mustache that curled up at the ends. He wore the traditional *keffiyah* wrapped around his head and rested his walking stick, made from the branch of an olive tree, against the wall. As he sat down, ancient dust and biblical sand billowed up from the folds of his caftan.

A cultured Romanian woman was nervous. Her veins were deep in her fleshy arms, but I managed to find a tiny blue one, hidden on the inner aspect of her pale forearm. When she smiled weakly in thanks to me, I noticed her bleeding gums and knew I would likely be transfusing her with platelets later that day.

Twenty-one-year-old Talia had completed her army service and had just been accepted to law school, but on a hiking trip in the Galilee with friends, after climbing Mount Gilboa she had noticed bruises along her arms and legs. She was diagnosed with a rare disease called aplastic anemia, a complete malfunction of the bone marrow, and only a transplant could save her life. Luckily, her sister was a close and willing match.

Yuri was an 18-year-old new immigrant who'd had to defer his army duty because of his illness. He was worried about the stigma of not serving in the army, but I heard Dr. Ben Cassis say privately that Yuri would probably not survive long enough to experience that stigma and would have to endure only the stigma of cancer. His parents tiptoed around him, speaking in Russian. Yuri translated for them and had his own questions, too. "What does 'white blood cell' mean? When will be my last day?" He was alarmed to overhear the doctor say that he had "no cells."

"What does that means, 'no cells'?" I explained that the chemotherapy had wiped out all his cells, good and bad, to the lowest possible level, called the nadir. This made him vulnerable to infection, but soon his bone marrow would begin to produce healthy cells that would protect him.

Later, Aviva reprimanded me. "Don't talk to patients so much, Tilda. Leave that to the doctor." But Hannah, who was the head nurse of the clinic, didn't mind what I did, though she preferred to offer patients warmth and affection rather than factual information. She was a petite, lively woman with a mane of wild, dark-blond hair, lots of jangling jewelry, and silver rings on her fingers. Hannah ran the clinic like the hostess of a cocktail

lounge, moving among the patients, chatting and laughing with families, offering advice, tea, and coffee, and
ensuring that everyone was comfy. She made her rounds
to each patient receiving chemo or a transfusion, offering
blankets, painkillers, or a clean vomit basin, and always a
kind, encouraging word.

"*Insh'allah*," she said to the Arab patients, invoking
God's mercy on their behalf. When patients vomited, she
rubbed their backs and told them, "That's great! Keep
going!" Even to the sickest patients, patients we knew
would likely die, Hannah said, "You're doing so well."

What a snow job! One day I challenged her. "Why do
you say it's going to be okay for them? Why give them
false hope? Shouldn't we be helping them accept reality?"

"There will be enough time for that," Hannah said.
"Right now, hope is just as important as chemotherapy—
maybe even more."

HANNAH EXPLAINED TO ME how our Arab patients
came to us. "The hospital bus brings them in the morning from the *occupied territories*," she started off, allowing
a few extra seconds for that contentious phrase to sink
into my brain. "They receive treatments and then the bus
returns them to their homes in Gaza or the West Bank."

Once, I looked out the window and saw a circle of
bedouin mothers eating their mid-morning meal of grapes,
pita bread, and sunflowers seeds. They lifted their veils
to spit out the seeds, and sat laughing and talking while
minding their children, who played all around them.

Hannah lit a cigarette. "They know their child is sick and can't get proper medical treatment in their villages, but they don't like to come to us. Slowly, they are gaining confidence in us, but if their village is put under curfew or they're hassled at the border after a terrorist attack, all is lost. Have you noticed how blood tests make them nervous? They're scared we'll take too much and they don't like getting Jewish blood. All in all, they're grateful but would rather not be dependent on us. Maybe one day we'll realize that disease is the enemy, not one another."

Aviva saw the situation differently. One morning at breakfast she spoke about an Israeli soldier who was killed in a terrorist attack on the northern border. One of his kidneys had been transplanted into a ten-year-old Arab boy in renal failure. "Don't you think we should take care of our own first?" she asked me, fuming.

"We must put all personal feelings aside," said Dr. Cassis, coming into the room and pouring himself a cup of coffee. He was a dark-skinned Moroccan Jew who dressed for work formally in a suit and tie that he removed the moment he walked out the door at the end of each day. He was brilliant, but stern and unapproachable. "What we do here is pure, untainted by politics. That's the beauty of medicine." It was unlike him to speak about the beauty of anything, and it stirred me to hear him say that.

ONE OF THE FIRST patients admitted to the bone-marrow transplant unit was a high-ranking army officer named Shaul Dayan. The treatment we had given him for his multiple myeloma was successful, but he still got infections and mouth sores. Even so, he looked virile and handsome. One morning Dr. Ben Cassis told me he wanted to perform a bone marrow biopsy on Shaul, so I began to gather everything he would need for the procedure. I rushed around, setting up as quickly as possible, as I could hear him pacing impatiently outside the door. I had to keep running in and out to retrieve things I'd forgotten and when I came back in, Shaul said, "Listen, don't let old Ben Cassis put pressure on you. This is what you will need for the procedure." He made me a list: gauze, sterile drapes, a *jamshidi* (a specialized instrument for performing the biopsy), a large syringe, and an assortment of glass slides and containers for the samples of his own bone marrow. "Relax," he told me, "you can do it."

Dr. Cassis performed the difficult procedure, which involved puncturing the hip bone with a large needle and extracting a sample of bone marrow. Most patients screamed during that test, but Shaul smiled. Assisting with this procedure always upset me, because I imagined how excruciating the patient's pain must be and I knew how much depended on the results.

After the biopsy, Dr. Cassis left the room abruptly and I stayed behind to tidy up. Shaul saw that I was distraught and put his arm around my waist to comfort me. I couldn't help but fall in love with him. In Shaul's case, that was a particularly easy thing to do, and I was not the only one susceptible to his charms. Rarely a day or night passed when there was not a beautiful woman at his bedside.

"I am his wife," said a woman.

"I am his girlfriend," said one on a separate occasion.

"I am his lover," said another.

"I am his commanding officer," said yet another.

"I am his wife," said a different one, and I didn't ask any questions.

Later that day, Dr. Cassis showed me the results of Shaul's bone marrow biopsy. "He's at his nadir," he said grimly. "He's vulnerable to infection. We'll have to put him in protective reverse isolation."

Now we had to approach Shaul in gowns, gloves, and masks. We were trying to protect him from organisms we might be harboring. Over the top of my mask, I smiled at him with my eyes and he smiled back with all of him. "Are you cold?" I asked. "Here's a blanket."

"Sit down," he said, "and be with me."

"Of course." I sat next to him on his bed. "I'm here. I'm with you."

"Breathe," he said, and we sat quietly for a few minutes. He handed me a pair of headphones and put on his, and plugged them both into his tape recorder. "Listen to this."

"It's magnificent," I said, still breathing for him.

"Of course it is," he grinned. "It's Bach's *Magnificat*." He lowered the volume. "Tilda, when two people listen to music together, it is an act more intimate than sex. Music is direct experience, the only one that two people can feel at the same time. Even during lovemaking each person is inside their own orgasm, experiencing their private pleasure. Only music can be felt simultaneously."

I was loath to change the subject, but I had to ask him something. "Shaul, are you afraid?"

He thought for a moment. "Not of death," he said, "only of pain."

ONE NIGHT I had another opportunity to work with Dr. Ben Cassis. I took over from the day nurse and she gave me report about Dawud, a 22-year-old man from Gaza, recently diagnosed with leukemia. He was coughing up blood and his blood pressure was low. Shortly after she left, I took my own reading and could barely detect it. His pulse was weak and thready. He was cool and clammy. I opened up his IV and let fluid pour in, then called Dr. Cassis at home and reported my findings.

"He's gone into septic shock," he said to me. "Damn it," he said to himself. He began to outline exactly what he wanted me to do: give lots of fluid, plus two units of packed red blood cells and ten units of platelets; start him on a different, stronger antibiotic and a drug I wasn't familiar with called dopamine.

"*Ya! Allah!*" cried the patient's young wife along with his mother and sisters, who gathered around his bed. "*Ya! Allah!*" they wailed and threw themselves upon his body. They had turned his bed around to face Mecca, in case he should die before the morning.

As I hung the first unit of blood, I looked up to see Dr. Ben Cassis walking in the door. For the rest of that night we worked side by side. I gave the antibiotics and assisted him as he inserted a central line into the patient's subclavian vein, through which I could run the dopamine faster and more safely. I took care of the other patients while he stayed with Dawud. At dawn, we took a break and sat down at the nurses' station. I thought about Aviva and what she'd say when she arrived in the morning. She would look at the mess and exclaim, "You made all this effort for a guy who might go on to bomb us?"

He looked at me and, as if reading my mind, said, "We must never hesitate." He raked his fingers through his dark hair. "The Arabs hate us and don't want us in the West Bank or the Gaza Strip. I dare say they don't want us in Tel Aviv or Haifa, either. The bottom line is that they don't want us here at all. However, we must have no hesitation whatsoever about what we do as doctors and nurses."

I got up to make us coffee and when I returned, I saw to my utter embarrassment that he was reading my journal, which I had accidentally left out on the desk at the nurses' station. Because he had opened it from right to left as he would a Hebrew book, he wasn't reading about my wild adventures and fantasies (many involving him) but rather from the few pages at the back where I kept a running list of the patients who had died, along with a few details to always remind me of each one.

"Why do you do this?" he asked sadly. To him it was a list of his failures.

"It's how I remember them," I explained. He looked at me. He stood up and drew me into his arms. I could feel his breath on my hair. "Oh, Tilda," he said in that ice-cream way they all had of saying my name. Then he kissed me. The thought of war and enemies so close by was such a turn-on that I wanted to stay in his arms as long as possible but within seconds, I felt the kiss melting away and the hug petering out.

I HAD BEEN in Israel almost a year to the day when I got home from work one evening to find a message on the answering machine from Pearl, my mother's caregiver. "Your mother is sick. She had a stroke and is in the hospital, but she is okay. God is love."

It was spring, and once again the sweet smell of the orange blossoms in the groves near the hospital filled the air. The cow-pasture hills were covered in wildflowers. Just as everything was coming into bloom, I had to tear myself away from it all and return to my dreary responsibilities back home. As I packed up to go, I thought back over the year. Talia was completely cured and in her first year of law school. Abdullah was in remission. Yuri was feeling great and came to visit us with his girlfriend to tell us they were engaged. Dawud made it through that difficult night, but died a few months later. Shaul was at home dealing with terrible bone pain. I didn't inquire about the others. I was leaving.

Ben Cassis said goodbye. "You are a fine young woman and an excellent nurse. I'm glad we didn't ruin you. We wish you well." But he must have known what I felt for him, because he tenderly touched my cheek as tears dripped down my face. He bent down to speak softly to me. "We're friends," he said, "and friendship is more important than love. Remember that."

A Midwife in Laos

~

Maribeth Diver, CNM, MSN

UNLIKE MOST Western *falang* (expatriates) living in Vientiane, Laos, we did not live downtown but in a village called Ban Nong Da, about 25 minutes away from the city. The unpaved road was filled with enormous pot-holes, but it was worth it to live right on the Mekong River. We had a tropical garden with banana and papaya trees and could look across the river to Thailand. We watched boats and fishermen, and families bathing in the twilight.

One day I was at a friend's house in a small part of the neighboring village. Little girls stood outside a tiny window looking up at me, and when I turned to look and smile at them, they laughed and laughed. When I didn't look at them, they waited patiently for me to turn again. We kept up this game and it kept all of us laughing.

Almost all of the little girls had naked babies strapped on their backs in colorful slings. I watched them casually help each other to readjust the babies and to retie a sarong when it came loose. I was in wonder at the ease with which these little mothers cared for their siblings, a normal part of every day. Some of them were as young as five or six, but they never seemed to struggle with the weight of even the chubbiest baby. I loved to see that the fathers and boys often carried babies in slings as well, and took as much joy in children as the women do.

Driving to work each day, I realized that the streets of Vientiane were one of my favorite things. The roads were chaos, a bevy of motorbikes, cars, and *tuk-tuks*, small motorized rickshaws, following no kind of law or logic that I could understand. Children and animals ran about, and carts loaded high with produce weaved their way through the bustle. Men on bikes sold sweet fruits and juices, and rang their bells over and over. Monks were everywhere, young and old, wearing traditional orange robes. The roads seemed to be the center of life. Houses, shop fronts, vendors, restaurants, and the colorful Buddhist temples (*wat* in the Lao language) lined their edges. There were simple square Lao houses of wood and bamboo, built on stilts so that most of daily life took place in the shade afforded below. There were also beautiful French colonial estates with formal gardens. There were many contrasts: rich and poor, lush and dusty, so busy and yet so simple. Each morning my mind raced and tried to wrap itself around the enigma that was Vientiane. And still today I can see it.

I'M ON MY little motorbike, wearing a *sihn*, the traditional long skirt, and a funny big helmet, being good-heartedly laughed at by everyone. A grandmother bathes a squealing child with a hose. A mama hen and her chicks nest in flowerpots by the side of the road. I see school kids walking in their uniforms, arm-in-arm. I see amazing feats: Lao families of five traveling on one motorbike, babies balanced on hips, toddlers standing on footrests. So many mutts nap on the roadside. They live lazily together with chickens and pigs and goats and all the grumpy roosters. There is always something aromatic cooking nearby, and there are brilliant fruits and vegetables at the simplest of markets. There is always noise and laughter in Laos.

And everywhere, there are babies and children, and all the animals have their young. It's easy to recall my earliest and most enduring impression of Laos: there are so, so many babies—human babies and animal babies. Little suckling pigs and puppies and sweet toddling goat kids, and baby water buffalo with swishing tails and chubby bare buns. Young calves, often twins, sleep in the shade below their mothers. Tiny chicks are everywhere. Geckos mate all over the walls every evening. The sheer fertility of this land is overwhelming. As I drive, I smile at all the LIFE. I'm sad to realize how empty and lonely our Western cities and neighborhoods are in contrast.

When I get to work, I enjoy my favorite moment of each day, beginning with walking into Mei le Dek (Mother and Child) Health Hospital, where I volunteer as a midwife. Though patients are not seen until 9:00 a.m., at

8:00 the halls are already bursting full, names on the long list to be seen. There are more pregnant bellies, nursing babies, and wide-eyed toddlers than I've seen in one place ever before; my eyes feast and my heart feels full. This very moment, this is what I've been waiting for!

LIKE MOST OF the Lao women, I wore a traditional skirt, and the women greeted me with big smiles, laughing to see a Westerner in Lao clothes. Every morning I was greeted by probably 100 *sabaidee ton saos*, salutations of good morning from the patients and the hospital staff. I'd found that people liked to touch white skin, and often women approached me just to do this, and to smile at me shyly. Every day I humbly relished these moments and was newly grateful for the opportunity of this experience.

I spent my first months in Vientiane, the capital city of Laos, looking for a paying job without success. The challenges that businesses faced in Laos were many, and for better or worse I'd come to understand that international aid programs and nongovernmental organizations are businesses no less than any other. The desperation I felt as a qualified and motivated midwife, willing to work for peanuts (and a visa), was so frustrating. I thoroughly expected to move here and be welcomed with open arms into the type of job I'd dreamed of and worked toward for years. It was nothing like this. There is so much need, especially in maternal-child health, but because of many political and economic difficulties not a lot was getting done.

Eventually I walked into Mei le Dek and politely insisted they let me volunteer. It took months to gain approval through the various levels of government bureaucracy, one ministry after another—to work for free. I am proud to know, however, that I am maybe the only non-Lao to get official approval from the Communist Lao government to work in a government hospital, without the affiliation of an aid program. This process was quite a learning experience in itself.

I tried to spend the months of waiting wisely, getting to know the Lao language and customs, enjoying some traveling, and trying to be involved in other ways. I had a great opportunity to tour seven district and provincial hospitals and health clinics, deep in the oldest part of Laos in the Khammoune Province.

I gave a presentation on infant and toddler nutrition to an international mothers' group. I did some short-term work for a large business, editing and revising a study that examined the health and nutritional indices and socioeconomic profiles of over 10,000 people from 311 villages. This work included statistical reanalysis of the data and extensive contact with local government ministries and agencies, and was a great learning experience in networking abroad.

Working at Mei le Dek was, in equal measures, both wonderful and challenging. My months there opened my eyes to why organizations require applicants to have international experience to apply. It's hard to understand how to work effectively when cultures vary so completely.

I made the newcomer's mistake of assuming that I could come in with all my grand ideals and big plans and make a difference—really save some mothers and babies!

I could not yet understand how difficult things were and how slowly things must change. I learned something essential to understand if you're interested in international health work: every single healthcare provider—especially midwives—holds fast to deep-rooted clinical beliefs and practices. And this is no less true for practitioners in underprivileged countries. Though many of the clinical practices were contrary to my deeply held midwifery beliefs, I had to remember: every good caregiver believes as wholly as I do that what he or she is doing is right. And the caregivers at Mei le Dek were dedicated to the women and babies they served and were doing the very best they could with very little at their disposal.

The problems began with outdated and impoverished medical and nursing education systems and grew greater with a serious lack of facilities and supplies and a lack of livable wages for the staff. The midwives, who worked 24-hour shifts, made the equivalent of ten U.S. dollars a month. The philosophies inherent to Lao people also presented unique differences. Laos is a Communist country with an almost exclusively Buddhist faith, which translated into a very strong focus on the moment-to-moment, an absence of planning for the future, and a natural avoidance of personal responsibility or individual accountability. By the nature of the system, there were many challenges.

My personal struggles were exacerbated by my limited language skills, my lack of funding or support from an outside source, my idealism, and my lack of professional experience. I moved to Laos just a week after sitting for my midwifery boards, and by the time I began volunteering at Mei le Dek it had been a year since I'd "caught a baby" and my confidence level was low.

Many of the midwives and doctors I met were highly experienced and therefore did not value what I first tried to offer them. I learned to focus on the little things, realizing that I did have a responsibility to help them with issues of practical safety and advancement of knowledge, but I did not have a right to try to influence their birthing or clinical philosophies. I also deeply appreciated that I learned from them every bit as much as they from me.

I was a foreigner, with a great education and access to all the latest evidence-based research, but I was not privileged to understand the subtleties of the population served. And that is imperative to effective caregiving!

Another major thing I learned during my job search: international health work by Westerners generally involves paperwork, albeit important paperwork, not hands-on care. Be prepared for this if you're interested in pursuing international midwifery. I designed a statistics program to track the hospital's utilization numbers and hope it can be used to track their health outcomes as well. So many interesting facts can be gleaned from this—for instance, I observed that "multips" (non-first-time mothers) often receive antenatal care at the hospital but don't come there for their births, and that parents bring in sick boys for medical care at a much higher rate than they bring in sick girls. I think that these insights can do a lot of good if put to work in program development.

A lot of my time was also spent providing what the staff expressed they wanted most from me: English-language and computer training. This was tons of fun, not to mention great for my Lao language skills. I also wrote proposals to liaison with local international health and development organizations, to help the hospital obtain needed funds and create some lasting affiliations. But that's an enormous project, and I hoped that without me this work would continue.

More than anything, the hospitals needed facilities and money. They had a few sinks but very limited cleaning supplies, and no training for the cleaning staff. After each birth they would wipe the floor with the same mop and bucket of water and put a new plastic drape over the bottom half of each delivery table. They didn't wipe the table or the stirrups, as there was nothing to wipe them with and no one to do the laundry. And the same waste bucket was propped under each woman's bottom for the birth.

The pregnant women had to bring everything they needed; if they didn't bring baby blankets, the father gave his shirt for the baby to be wrapped in. The postpartum wards were three rooms with 15 women in each. The rooms were crowded with up to 45 women and their many family members, including young children. The families slept on mats on the floor beside their mothers, sisters, daughters, or friends. They stayed to give comfort care and to provide all food, as the hospital provided none. For the bleeding new mothers and all these visitors, there were only three toilets.

Clinically, I held antenatal clinic two days a week and worked in the delivery room the rest of the time. There were many joyous births, and sad ones too; there were normal births, but also some very sick mothers and babies. I learned some great tricks and shared knowledge with the staff. I was privileged to conduct prenatal and postpartum visits at home for friends and neighbors near my home, and I learned much about the fascinating traditions a new Lao mother must follow after birth.

Newly birthed mothers both sleep and sit over hot burning coals, as it is believed that the warmth cleans and purifies their wombs. The temperature may be 100 degrees with 100 percent humidity, but for a week or two they "roast" themselves around the clock. Mothers generally place a large knife or sword under their bedding or their pillows. When women go outside to use the restroom, their husbands stay with them and hold this knife aloft. They believe that the knife wards off evil spirits who seek to harm either the mother or the new baby.

New mothers in Laos also follow an extremely strict postpartum diet. For several weeks they mostly eat white chicken, white rice, and a strong tea. There are strongly held beliefs that eating an improper food might render the mother infertile in the future. It would be especially devastating to eat an egg: it could mean that the woman would have no future eggs herself. After six weeks there will be a *bac*, the traditional blessing ceremony, for the baby, hosted by a high-ranking monk. The mother and baby will have their wrists layered with hundreds of pieces of plain white string. Friends and family tie the strings on while reciting a blessing, and often tuck money between the threads. It was a great privilege to learn about these fascinating traditions and beliefs.

There were some hardships to balance out the joy of all these special moments: struggles with miscellaneous stomach viruses and thousands of mosquito bites. When the brown waters of the Mekong River flooded our house, I chased out frogs for weeks. And there were many days without power or running water. My boyfriend had a bout with typhus fever, and we lost a beloved dog to a mystery virus.

Lao people were so curious about Westerners that our English friend had a neighbor who sat in a tree to watch how our friend spent each evening. Laotians were indeed as curious as this and were lovers of gossip. News of our activities and routines quickly spread through our village. We relished this as a special part of the experience of living immersed in another culture. And the kindness and generosity of the Lao people opened my heart in new and joyous ways.

Susy

~

Sue Averill, RN, MBA, and *Elizabeth Coulter, RN*

ALL EYES WATCHED the fine crimson streak that followed the surgeon's scalpel as he traced it across the woman's swollen belly. Immediately, the Finnish nurse jumped in and said the opening he made was not big enough to pull a mouse through, let alone a baby. He hesitated, and she nodded for him to continue. He carved a beautiful line. After all, the 75-year-old doctor was a plastic surgeon, not an obstetrician.

When I look back, the moment had the makings of a bad joke: a retired plastic surgeon, a general practitioner, an anesthesiologist, and three nurses traveled to Guatemala for a plastic surgery mission and ended up doing a C-section. In the punch line there would be a talking duck, but all we saw were Guatemalan roof dogs—scary-looking mongrels who barked from the flat rooftops—and none of those spoke English.

We were exhausted from an arduous 14-hour trip in the old, battered trucks that bounced around on the washed-out roads that ran north, through the mountains. The thin vinyl seats offered little padding over the large metal springs, which jabbed with every jolt from the ruts beneath the tires. Several times we'd give a communal gasp as the truck slid dangerously close to the road's edge. The driver would laugh nervously and say, "Okay, okay," then lean forward and squint to see through the pounding rain on the windshield.

Hour after hour, we climbed above tree lines, passing graveyards on hillsides with tombs painted in bright colors so God would see them and lift the souls to heaven. I'd long given up on finding a comfortable position and accepted being jostled until my chattering teeth hurt, when finally, in the mist of the far northern highlands, we'd reached our destination: a small town called Barillas.

The people of Barillas have lived in isolation for generations, so our arrival did not go unnoticed. They are descendants of the Mayans, with coarse black hair that frames round faces, and are short in stature. I literally stood head and shoulders above the men and women who welcomed us.

As the only Spanish-speaking member of the team, I translated as local men helped us unpack our supplies and equipment. We had brought everything needed for the slight, white-haired surgeon to work his magic on cleft palates and lips and to graft burned skin. An old man directed me to the flat concrete house that would act as our home base. As I walked past a group of women and children who'd gathered to stare, I untied my long blond hair and let it fall over my shoulders. On a previous mission to Pakistan, I had learned that my hair could be a bridge to the women. They loved to touch and braid it.

The supplies were placed against the wall of the meagerly furnished living area. The unpacking could wait until morning. Our aching bodies needed a warm shower and soft bed but before I could even open my backpack, the door opened and a small woman walked in. I asked her to slow her rapid speech so I could understand. I nodded as she emphasized each word with hand gestures. Finally, the Finnish nurse could stand it no longer.

"What is she saying?" she said in her thick accent.

"She is the local midwife," I answered. "And she wants us to deliver a baby by C-section."

A young woman had been in labor for more than 18 hours and was becoming exhausted. The town's only doctor had left months ago for a vacation and never returned. The midwife smiled and turned to the surgeon.

"Doctor," she said, pointing to the two tired men, who looked at each other with concern.

Wearily, the five of us followed the midwife down the muddy path to the young woman's house. Along the way, the general practitioner mentioned that he hadn't seen a delivery since med school, 20 years prior. The plastic surgeon let out a nervous laugh and told him to multiply that time period by two and a half. The two other nurses could offer little support; one specialized in geriatrics, and the other was an operating-room director. As for myself, a typical emergency-room nurse, I would rather walk barefoot across burning coals than face a pregnant woman who says she needs to push. But the moment we entered the home and saw the young woman sitting on a wing-backed chair, drenched in sweat and panting through a contraction, we forgot about our own fears.

I crouched beside the young woman and placed a cool washcloth on her forehead. Using my softest voice, I introduced her to the members of the team. She peered through half-closed eyes and moaned. The GP approached her with the confidence of a doctor, and placed his hands on her abdomen to determine that the baby's position was, fortunately, head down. "At least I think I felt a head," he whispered to the surgeon as I translated his encouraging findings to the girl's mother-in-law. A pelvic exam revealed her cervix was only 3 centimeters dilated and that she had a very small pelvis. If she was lucky, the baby would be tiny enough to pass through.

The doctors huddled as I stroked the young woman's hair and whispered words of encouragement. At 19, her life had already been determined. She would be a mother and take care of her family. There were no other options. Her mother-in-law fussed about, offering sips of water and stroking her shoulder gently. I asked about the young woman's husband and was told he worked night shift at the local coffee factory.

The decision was that we would let her labor during the night and hope—with fingers and toes crossed—that nature would take its proper course. In the meantime, we would return to our rooms and rest. The Finnish nurse said she would have the OR ready to go, just in case.

I was asleep the moment my head hit the pillow.

The knock on the door came even before the roosters had a chance to crow. I leaped out of bed, shivering as I tiptoed barefoot over the cold linoleum. It was the midwife.

"Susanna," she said to me. "She needs help."

The midwife chattered as we rushed to the young woman's house. Three hours ago her membranes had ruptured, and she had been in hard labor since. At that time, her contractions were two minutes apart and her cervix was fully effaced, (shortened), and 9 centimeters dilated (opened). And that's where she stayed. Stuck.

The young woman was leaning forward, her head resting on a table, when we entered the house. Her mother-in-law pulled on my arm, pleading with me to help. The young woman's husband sat in the corner, waiting. She barely acknowledged my presence as she breathed through another contraction. Watching her made me realize how soft our culture had become, remembering how people sauntered into the ER, snapping gum and crunching Doritos, claiming ten out of ten on the pain scale, all the while talking on their cell phones.

I waited for a break between contractions, then instructed the husband to carry his wife to our transportation. He placed her in the bed of a neighbor's pickup truck before she screamed in pain with another contraction. I jumped in the back and held her in my arms as the neighbor drove to the clinic.

It wasn't a delivery room, but a bare eight-by-ten-foot concrete room that was going to be our OR "suite." A steel gurney, antique by our standards, would be our delivery bed. I looked for a crank or pump to elevate the head of the gurney, but there was none. I placed a pillow under the woman's left hip so the baby would get more blood flow, and folded a blanket for beneath her head.

The team anesthesiologist positioned her on her side as he prepared to introduce a catheter for spinal anesthesia. I found a broom and began to sweep out rainwater that had overflowed into the room during the night. A wet floor would short out the cautery machine, which would be needed to stop any bleeding during the C-section. With the pain controlled by the spinal, the woman relaxed. She didn't flinch when I started the IV and placed a Foley catheter into her bladder. Half a liter of urine filled the catheter bag. I wondered whether her full bladder had impeded her labor.

The surgeon—plastic surgeon, that is—entered the room with the GP at his side. A drape blocked the patient from seeing the first, gentle cut of the scalpel. I stood beside her head and offered reassurance. The doctor tested the cautery, an electrical device used to apply heat to blood vessels to stop or decrease bleeding, and realized the power outlet in the room didn't work. To control the oozing blood, he placed clamps on the edges of the incision. In the meantime, the caretaker of the clinic found an extension cord and ran it over the floor into the room. The connection sparked as the machine was plugged in, so we gave up on cautery.

"You can't even pull a mouse out of that," the Finnish nurse said, pulling off the clamps the GP had meticulously placed. "She's not going to bleed to death—you'll never get a baby out with these on!"

The surgeon extended the length of the incision as I continued to talk with the young woman, repeatedly answering her questions the same way.

"Everything is okay," I said, over and over.

The scalpel cut into the thick wall of the uterus. I was thankful for acting skills gained in high school theater courses that allowed me to keep a calm face as I watched the urine in the catheter bag turn bright red. The surgeon must have nicked her bladder. When the incision was wide enough, he tentatively slid his gloved hand into the patient's belly. He was feeling around, shaking his head, when the Finnish nurse grabbed his hand and pushed it in deeper.

"Cradle the baby in your hand," she said. "Then you can scoop it out. Just like a melon ball."

The surgeon tugged on the baby's body and head, but nothing budged. The GP placed his hand beneath the drape and pushed up. Still, the baby's head was engaged deep in the pelvis. The surgeon looked over his mask at the GP, who looked at the Finnish nurse, who looked at me. I looked at the young woman's trusting brown eyes. I distracted her as the GP placed his fist in the birth canal and pushed. The baby popped out into the surgeon's cupped hands and began to wail. A six-pound, five-ounce girl.

After the infant was warmed beneath a gooseneck lamp, mother and baby were settled into the overnight stay room. Unlike in American hospitals, where there are strict visiting policies, mother and baby had a stream of visitors, ladies of the local community who had heard about the delivery. The day continued with the surgeon happily back in his comfort zone of repairing gaping lips and mouths. I held kids as they woke up from their surgeries and passed them to nervous parents who were praising God for miracles.

During my first mid-morning break, I decided to check on my obstetrical patient. I walked into the room crowded with women and children, all talking and laughing. The moment I said hello, conversations stopped and laughter ceased as all eyes stared at me. My five-foot-nine-inch frame towered over them, and with my fair skin, blue eyes, and long blond hair, I must have looked like something out of a storybook.

I smiled and greeted the teenager who was now a mother. She passed the squirming bundle to me. I held her little brown face beside mine.

"Look!" I proclaimed. "She looks just like me!"

The room erupted in laughter and as I returned the

baby to her mother, many nodded and smiled in agreement. As the day progressed, the joke traveled around the women in the community. The little brown-eyed, black-haired baby was the spitting imagine of the tall blond American nurse named Sue.

The young mother's recovery was unremarkable, and the baby did great. She was discharged two days after the surgery, needing only a handful of Tylenol for post-op pain. Before leaving, she asked that I convey her thanks to the surgeon. She knew that without his skills, the baby would have died inside her and she would have died as well. I nodded and hugged her and her husband, whose face beamed when he held his little daughter. I asked him what they were going to name the child. Grandma held the baby next to me and said, "She looks like you. Her name is 'Susy.'"

The week progressed quickly. Between our surgical cases, people came to us with varying medical needs. Our team really did become the town's doctors, caring for boils and lacerations and a child who had been unconscious for hours after being kicked in the forehead by a horse. Dozens of children had their deformities exchanged for hugs and thanks and tears. I knew the life-changing impact our team had on these children and wondered how we could teach that a prenatal vitamin, high in folic acid, would prevent many of these disfigurements.

Three years had passed before I had a chance to return to Barillas, this time with a pediatrician friend to do screening for an upcoming surgical mission. Very little had changed in the village since I had last visited it, and news of *"gringas"* caused a stir in the local population. On the second day of our work, the midwife came with a lunch invitation from Susy's family.

Susy was sleeping in the bedroom when we arrived. The living area was filled with relatives and neighbors wanting to meet the renowned American "Sister Susana." I instantly recognized the young mother, who hugged me and immediately pulled down her skirt to show me her C-section scar. Only two inches long, it had healed so well it was barely noticeable.

"The other women are jealous," she said as she scooped rice onto my plate. "They want that doctor to come back for when they have babies."

I doubted the surgeon, now nearing 80, would be interested in revitalizing his career in obstetrics. It was easy to laugh about the event now, but at the time it had been terrifying. As we chatted and drank delicious local coffee, a little girl appeared in the doorway, rubbing her sleepy eyes with her hands.

Amid a room filled with black-haired, brown-eyed, bronze relatives stood a fair-skinned little moppet of blond curls and bluegreen eyes—little Susy. She ran over to me, put her warm hand in mine, looked up, and smiled.

PART TWO

In the Shadows

Waterlife

~

John B. Fiddler, RN, ANP

Eastern chad, july 2007: I find myself standing in a sandy clearing on the edge of what looks like a
lake. The water is dilute chocolate milk. Across the water
on the far bank, I see women and children wading and
washing clothes. Behind them a gentle slope leads up to a
village of traditional grass huts and the white tarpaulins
of refugee shelters. Our Land Cruisers have just emerged
from a grove of palm trees, and two rafts of empty oil
drums lashed together are anchored to the bank and sit
waiting. Above, birds with curved beaks circle and call.
Our two cars are parked, spattered with drying mud, the
engines clicking as they cool down after the journey. We
can drive no farther. This wadi is impassable and will be
from now until November; we are all just glad to have
made it this far. The waters are rising fast, and we have to

make the crossing without delay. Our destination: Kerfi, a bustling market town 45 kilometers south of Goz Beida, the regional capital of the Ouaddai province, which forms part of the border with Sudan.

Watching us is a crowd of boys and some men. The boys seem to be smaller than their American counterparts for their ages, which I guess to be from six to 13 years. Most regard us with some curiosity but generally appear unimpressed by our arrival. They are thin, but strong and healthy looking. Their skin is patterned with dust or slick from the water. Some are chewing on the kernels of a coconut-like fruit from the palm trees that splits open to reveal a bright orange pulp. This splash of color in a semidesert landscape makes for an unforgettable first impression. Momentarily, for me, the year 2007 ceases to exist; the ancient African past and the present become one.

It is hot here, so for six months of the year the waters become a cooling playground for these children. The water serves also as laundry, toilet, and garbage disposal, and is often the only water available to drink. It is also home and breeding ground for some of the most insidious illnesses we will encounter, including the great killer, malaria. Our arrival noted, the kids resume playing and swimming. As we set off on the slow-moving rafts for the far shore, the boys dive-bomb us from the trees, laughing and screaming as they attempt to wet us. Today they are invincible.

Chad is my second assignment with Doctors Without Borders. I worked in Burundi for ten months in 2005; there were no wadis there. Up to this point I have only read about these riverbeds and hollows that are easily crossed on foot in the dry season, then turn to impassable milky torrents during the rainy season. Now I am going to spend most of the next six months completely surrounded by them.

Around Kerfi, the local population converges on the town every Wednesday for a sprawling market that serves as a center of commerce and community. On market day, visitors will also take the opportunity to seek medical care. The village has a well-constructed but barren clinic manned by four government staff who are minimally trained as health aides. There are no doctors. My role here, then, is multifold. I am tasked to supervise the facility and assist the government staff with training and teaching. Our team also brings essential medications and will establish a pharmacy program. I will run a nutrition program and coordinate primary healthcare needs for a diverse population, including an influx of internally displaced persons forced from their homes close to the border with Sudan. These IDPs are the victims of new and old tribal conflict and ongoing war, and are the main reason we have decided to establish a presence here.

In the rainy season, sickness here increases, mortality increases, and anyone seriously ill is effectively trapped. I look at the village looming closer and ask myself what on earth I am doing here. I am thousands of miles from New York City and my 21st-century critical care unit with its high-tech modern equipment and fully stocked shelves. I'm used to having experts and laboratories just a call away. Will I be able to provide high-quality care here with the limited resources? Will I be able to use my assessment skills as a new nurse practitioner? How will I be able to diagnose exotic diseases that I have seen only in books? I realize the answers will surely find me. I won't be going anywhere for a while.

There is no situation quite as overwhelming for a medical caregiver as encountering your first crowd of waiting patients in an African clinic. The majority are women and children, almost always accompanied by a chorus of crying babies. These are the most vulnerable and are also the first ones to sicken. I am nervous beginning my first triage rounds, walking through the assembled patients, seeking those particularly ill who need to be seen first. Any child or adult with a fever (a cardinal sign of malaria) is automatically chosen and tested with a paracheck. This finger-prick test is rapid, and specific for malaria. If positive, this is immediately an indication for treatment.

In every new field assignment, I learn to negotiate situations so that the sickest patient is cared for first. I soon learn that in Kerfi, a sick baby or mother is not necessarily a priority. Triage does not apply quite as I understand it. One soon realizes that the local tribal chieftain, or the local military commander (and there are many of each), may take priority. Men also expect to be seen immediately and are uncomfortable waiting with females. We have to find a way to satisfy this population or no one will come to the clinic. We settle on the idea of making two separate waiting areas, one for women and children, the other for men. We triage women and children first, and then sit with the men and consult with them. We alternate between the two groups. This seems to work!

One particular tribal leader, swathed in a turban and dark glasses, walks into the clinic, pulls up his robe, turns his ample buttock toward me, and motions for an injection even though we have not even diagnosed an illness. Apparently he had received an injection some time before and liked the result. I learn that many in the community see injections as an efficacious, almost magical treatment. They do not think tablets or oral medications really work. I realize that I am being taught unexpected lessons. To try and address the misinformation and rumors, I must organize community outreach and education. I learn, too, that some patients who receive prescribed medicine take all the tablets at once. Perhaps they think it will work better? After my initial surprise that they are still standing ("you took all twenty of the pills I gave you at the same time?"), I plan to do teaching at the pharmacy to help ensure better understanding and compliance.

Apart from women, crying babies, and pushy chieftains, there is another population that presents at the clinic that intrigues me: the same-age children I see swimming at the banks of the wadi. They are mostly boys, but there are a handful of girls. They wait, hesitant and shy, eyes held to the ground. Through an interpreter I learn they have nonspecific symptoms such as abdominal pain or nausea. My colleague who is familiar with schistosomiasis, a water-borne infection endemic among children in this part of Africa, teaches me the critical diagnostic question to ask these patients: what is the color of their urine? Almost always uncomfortably, they reply "pink." We have our diagnosis. Another lesson learned. The parasite that infects the children is contracted from the water while swimming; it eventually anchors in the bladder and produces a hematuria—blood in the urine. This disease can progress and can lead to serious chronic illness as the children grow up. If they grow up.

I grow sensitive to these patients. As a result, our team develops yet another simple parallel triage system. We put aside the children until there is a group of six or more; then we take them together to be weighed and registered. The children stand in a line, traipse into our pharmacy room where they each take a one-time dose of praziquantel, and trot off into the distance—most surely to swim and play in the microbe-laden water again.

These children quickly learn my name. As I walk the path back to our base at day's end, now no longer shy, they shout out, "Jon, Jon, Jon!" to grab my attention. In the clinic, the colorful, chaotic crowds of mothers and babies demand most of my attention. The older children are already considered the survivors; they have made it past the vulnerable times and with any luck have developed a protective immunity to some diseases. You tend to regard them as invulnerable, as perhaps they do themselves.

One day at the clinic I was called to one of the consultation rooms to see a sick child. He was about ten years old. He was lying on a crude bed frame close to the ground. Beside the bed his mother was on her knees holding his hand, mute with worry. The boy was breathing erratically, moaning, unresponsive, and drooling, his eyes rolled back in his head. We were pretty sure he had cerebral malaria, and while a nurse pricked his finger to test for this, we were already putting in an IV. I demanded a quick history of his illness. "Has he been sick long?" The translator told me he had been playing and swimming the day before. We attempted to inject some dextrose to correct hypoglycemia (low blood sugar) but even as we tried to save him, I knew it was too late. Pink foam started pouring from his mouth. It looked as though someone had shaken a bottle of cherry soda inside him. It was the ominous sign of pulmonary edema. Increased pressure in the blood vessels of his lungs had forced fluid into the air sacs, preventing them from absorbing oxygen. One of the nurses cautioned me not to tell the mother her son would die, as is my nursing instinct—"this is not done here." So I stood there and watched him dying as his mother sat beside him, distraught. I have never felt so helpless. Time stood still in this moment as an African future was slowly extinguished.

That night I, and other members of our team, went to bed extra early before the mosquitoes began their hungry dance at dusk. I wrapped myself in my mosquito net and closed my eyes. The bright color images of turbans, smiles, grimaces, and lives reeled past. In America, I have often heard it said that it is not natural for parents to outlive their children; it is not natural for parents to bury their own child. I write in my diary, "What do they know? It happens here all the time."

Four hundred and ninety-seven days later in New York City, the images of the hundreds of patients we served daily still dance brightly in my mind. I save the most tender feelings for those boys and girls—full of laughter—swimming in the waters of the wadis, then shyly presenting for treatment at the clinic. The survivors. The invincibles. I wonder what the future holds for them. I wonder how they are now and whether anything has changed. Then I realize—I have to go back. I still hear them calling my name. They have more to teach me.

T Girl

~

Sue Averill, RN, MBA

SHE CAME at the end of another hot, humid day when even a sip of water instantly erupted onto our skin as sticky, smelly sweat. We'd learned that if you don't drink, you don't sweat, although the nurse in me wondered how our kidneys were faring. With an exhausted sigh and a stretch of cramped muscles, I finished my line of 100 patients in the crumbling structure of Kakata Internally Displaced Persons (IDP) camp and glanced toward the entranceway. There was a thin, ragged child lying unconscious on a straw mat on the filthy concrete floor. Her breathing was rapid and shallow, and not a sound came from her parted cracked lips.

Fighting in Liberia's civil war to oust President Charles Taylor had mostly stopped by the end of 2003, but by that time, many of the country's population of three million had moved into IDP camps around the capital of Monrovia.

In February of 2004, I was one of three nurses sent by Northwest Medical Teams to provide consultations and medical care to six of these camps for a month. I was a 25-year veteran of various emergency departments in the Seattle/Tacoma area and had been involved in volunteer work for about five years, but never in Africa, never for this long, and never doing this type of work.

These medical clinics consisted of me and Heather, a nurse practitioner working in women's health in Seattle, sitting at one plastic table. Lois, a nurse from California, and a Liberian nurse sat at another. Inside and outside the "clinic"—either a stick-and-mud hut constructed for our use or a crumbling relic of an old concrete building like the one at Kakata—were lines of hundreds of patients, their families, and some camp residents who came for the pure entertainment value of white-skinned, blue-eyed foreigners. The noise levels were headache-producing within minutes of our arrival.

Another child whispered above the cacophony, "She is T Girl." They had played together the day before. Now her skin was feverishly hot, lips and conjunctiva (the thin membrane that covers the surface of the inner eyelid) showed the paleness of severe anemia, and she was unresponsive to voice or touch. I gently palpated her abdomen and couldn't understand what I felt—a hard, right-angle drop that went from the bottom of her breastbone to her pelvis. When Heather came rushing over, we looked at each other and said in unison, "Spleen?" I had never felt a spleen before, much less one that felt like the edge of a shelf.

Each clinic was packed with people whose problems we had no ability to diagnose—no testing, no labs, no X-ray, no textbooks—no idea.

"My skin can be HOT!" was the chief complaint.

Did that mean fever from malaria, with no way to test for it, and against which the available medications have a 50 to 75 percent resistance? Or was it yellow fever, as we'd heard reported here? Trauma? Another infection of some sort, perhaps elephantiasis (a mosquito-borne parasitic disease caused by tiny, threadlike worms that live in the human lymph system, best known from dramatic photos of people with grossly enlarged or swollen arms and legs)? Or polio, malnutrition, measles, schistosomiasis (a parasite that penetrates the skin of persons who are wading, swimming, bathing, or washing in contaminated water)—so many diseases we don't see in the United States! Without a doctor, a tropical medicine text, or appropriate medications and referral options, we felt lost, alone, and impotent to help these people. We had only each other.

English may be the national language of Liberia, but between the accent, gestures, and idioms, I was routinely bewildered. Translations took a moment to grasp. "When last you saw the moon?" meant "When was your last period?"; "water from the fish" referred to vaginal discharge; and "got belly" meant "pregnant."

People's names were nearly as confusing, with Young Boy (who might be 60), God Knows, Baby Doe, Darling Girl, and my favorite of favorites: Bacteria. We were provided "translators" at each camp, who mostly repeated our exact words while shouting directly in the face of the non-astonished patient.

A translation earlier that day had put us into fits of giggling. To my right, Heather was attempting to interview a mother about an infant in arms:

"Is the child breastfeeding?" Heather asked.

Blank stare.

"Will the baby eat?" she asked, tapping her own breast.

Blank stare.

"Does the child take milk?" Heather asked, as she pointed to the mother's exposed breasts.

Blank stare.

"She drinks?" Heather asked.

Blank stare.

The translator, an old man from the camp management, stuck his face in the mother's and at the exact moment when all noise miraculously stopped, shouted, "HE SUCK THE TITTY GOOD?" Mama turned to Heather and nodded.

Fruitlessly, we searched for T Girl's parents to give consent and accompany us; helpful residents ran off in different directions. The wait was excruciating; we knew that every minute we delayed, her chances of survival dropped precipitously. After what seemed like an hour, but was probably ten minutes, we finally agreed that her teen sister could accompany us for the two-hour drive to the hospital on the outskirts of the city. I thought of starting an IV, but to what purpose? Fluids alone would not save this child. We had no ability to diagnose, much less treat, and no medicines to give her even with a proper diagnosis.

We gathered up the other three or four ill babies and moms, piled our supplies on top of the white Toyota Land Cruiser, symbol of nongovernmental organizations around the world, and drove off with T Girl in my arms in the front seat, with Peter driving and Heather wedged around the gearshift.

Peter cautiously drove as fast as possible, avoiding the myriad piles of broken asphalt, potholes, broken-down vehicles, transport trucks with sacks of charcoal piled 30 feet in the air and workers sitting atop, bicycles, and women walking with bundles on their heads, weaving the vehicle through crowded markets until we were within minutes of the hospital.

T Girl seized. Not violently, not urgently, not with one of the tongue-biting, incontinent grand mal seizures we see in the emergency room. She seized with a gentle, upward-gazing, rhythmic twitching for several minutes. I cradled her in my arms and cheek-to-cheek softly talked into her ear, quietly singing and assuring her she was with friends. Heather and I locked eyes in that unspoken language of like minds, knowing the truth of the situation and what was to come. Heather moved shoulder-to-shoulder with me, arm supporting my arm, T Girl's head joining us together to

block her sister's view and that of the other backseat passengers so they would not become frightened.

I felt the soft warmth of her urine soak my scrubs. Her
pupils dilated and her twitching eased. She stopped breathing. She had died in my arms, ten minutes before arrival
at the hospital. I continued to rock T Girl and sing softly,
with Heather's arms supporting both of us. We could do
no more than console the silently weeping teen sister and
wrap the small body in a clean white sheet, promising to
take her back to Kakata Camp in the morning.

I've tried to look back at the emotions of the time, but
all are shrouded in tears and shame and grief. Children in
my world don't play with other kids one day and die the
next. Children in my world have access to medical care,
medical tests, medicines, and doctors. Children in my
world have abundant nutritious food to eat and schools
and clean clothes and homes to live in and parents who
were not killed in a civil war. Children in my world don't
live in eight-by-eight-foot mud-and-straw huts in IDP
camps, drink dirty water, or eat whatever food is brought
by an aid agency once a month. Children in my world
don't die in my arms, with me impotent to offer more
than mumbled assurances that they were among friends.
Forty-two million people are currently displaced from
their homes by war.

Forty-two million T Girls.

Since then I've worked four six-month missions with
Médecins Sans Frontières in Darfur, northern Uganda,
western Ethiopia, and South Sudan; and helped found

One Nurse at a Time, a nonprofit organization dedicated to assisting nurses enhance the nursing profession as they look for opportunities to serve locally, nationally, and internationally.

I ask myself now, with all the knowledge I've gained since then: What could I or should I have done differently for T Girl? Would different action on my part have had a different impact on that one child's life? What if I had been more prepared? I still don't know the answer to those questions, but T Girl brought me to commit my life to humanitarian nursing.

I Am Still Here

~

Connie Nunn, RN, BN

NEXT TO MY PICTURE in my high-school year-book it says, "Connie wants to become a nurse and work with CUSO." I discovered this note 15 years after I wrote it. I was 30 when I found this note while I, believe it or not, was preparing for my trip to Sierra Leone with CUSO, a group known as Canadian University Sewick Overseas, that sends volunteers overseas, as a nurse.

I had completely forgotten that I had the idea so early on. Where the seed was originally planted, I don't know, but it must have lingered in the back of my mind until I eventually took the leap and signed up. And as soon as I did, the idea quickly took root and kept me going from one field assignment to the next, from Sierra Leone to Ghana, Tajikistan, Pakistan, South Sudan, and Darfur, where I live today.

When I first left for Sierra Leone, my exposure to the developing world was limited to a two-and-a-half-week safari in Kenya, which I won through my nursing union in Montreal. It was a tourist safari, one where you drive around and look at animals, so it was not a developing-world experience at all.

My family was supportive of my decision, but they did not understand it because they did not know anybody who did international relief work. I think my colleagues at work thought it was weird, but they covered it up well with a beautiful red-leather passport holder as my parting gift. And perhaps it *is* weird. I can say that international nursing certainly is not for everybody. You have to accept that things are completely different from home, and adapt. Oftentimes, in countries like Sierra Leone where there was war, things can feel completely upside-down, but somewhere in the chaos you have to use your basic nursing skills and help people find ways to deal with at least some of their health issues. Therein lies your sense of order and purpose.

My wake-up call to this adaptation came within the first two weeks of my arrival in Sierra Leone. I was sent to a village with a local woman to the women's society bush—a secret society where girls go through different rites of passage to become women. My assignment was to teach traditional midwives in the secret society bush about clean deliveries and about maternal and child care.

Midwifery was not part of my nursing education, but I was given a little book in English with six scenarios

in which you would refer women to hospitals, four danger signs of pregnancy, and three arguments about why
people should go to health clinics. I had nothing to do
but read aloud from this little book, while a local—and
untrained—midwife translated. As I went on, I sensed
that she was not translating what I said, but rather giving
her own lecture on whatever she thought she should say.
After years of practicing public health in these environ-
ments, I now know that that is exactly what she did.

To the side of the midwives were young initiates,
teenage girls who had just been circumcised. They would
live in the bush for a few months, would receive guid-
ance from the society elder woman on being a good wife
and mother, and then would marry and have children.
The girls sat with their legs locked tightly together, their
faces covered in clay. I thought about the circumcision,
the excruciating pain they must have gone through, and
then about the potential problems that could develop.

I could not take the circumcision back, but I could
offer simple solutions if some of the girls started to have
problems. I advised the midwives to examine them and
prepare sitz baths, bowls of warm water, which the girls
could sit in if they had any complications. We also coun-
seled the midwives on antenatal care, such as administer-
ing tetanus toxoid vaccinations during the pregnancy. This
protects the baby from tetanus, which, until recently, killed
approximately 10 percent of newborns in Sierra Leone.

It was in this moment, while I was teaching midwifery with my perception of life and the universe in

this completely foreign environment, that the limitations, purpose, and gravity of international medical work settled in. It was 1980.

My work with CUSO also challenged the way in which I—and the programs in which I worked—interacted with others. CUSO provided medical care through a mission hospital that had been there for 30 years. One would think its history would make the hospital an unchallenged establishment in the community, but then a faith healer moved into town.

The faith healer's name was Haja, a title that means that she had been to Mecca on a pilgrimage. She set up camp at the opposite end of town from our hospital. She specialized in neurological problems and traveled with an entourage who organized the services and collected money. Her following exploded. Cars from neighboring countries, including Liberia and Guinea, would line up in this very rural village to receive care from Haja.

We were perplexed. How could a faith healer be taking all of our patients? The director of the hospital sent staff to observe Haja and how she interacted with her patients.

Looking back, this was the director's attempt to teach the hospital staff that the patients need to believe in the care they are receiving. Because hospital care can be impersonal and the staff sometimes uncaring, patients could not believe that they were receiving help, even if the medicines and treatment worked. This made room for faith healers like Haja, who may not be able to solve the problem medically but do make people believe they are being cared for because of the healer's personal interaction with them.

Because she failed to heal people within two months, confidence in the faith healer waned. As a result, her practice dried up,, confirming the strong connection between what people believe and where they seek care. For us, that meant that we needed to be more personal, more caring, so that the local people believed in the treatment they were receiving.

Traditional healers are something that I have encountered throughout my work in the developing world. The practices vary greatly. Some listen to the patient's problems and write a religious script on a piece of paper that is believed to cure the ailment when the patient eats it. There are faith healers, like Haja, who cure their followers by laying their hands on them. And then there are diviners who figure out who caused the illness and then demand that the patient pay money or perform a certain ritual to expel the sickness from the village. In the most extreme cases, the alleged source is expelled for the community, oftentimes with nowhere to go or anyone to turn to for support.

These are all beliefs that coexist with modern medicine in these countries. That's why public education and outreach is so important and something that International Medical Corps focuses on with every mission. These healers are a part of the cultural framework and you have to work with them, as well as the with village elders, community leaders, and government officials, so that Western medicine is accepted.

Sometimes, in countries like Sierra Leone and Sudan where there is war, it can be incredibly difficult to identify effective community leaders. As populations are displaced, so is the leadership structure. While leaders are appointed in the new resettlements areas, the people may recognize their former leader, not the one they inherit. Or there will be multiple leaders in one area for different groups of people who settled there.

With displacement, the mechanisms for choosing leaders are also in complete disarray. The rules are open, causing some leaders to be seen as illegitimate or forced. People often do not recognize these leaders, making the system even more decentralized and complicated. As a health worker, it is very hard to deal with and solve community health issues when there is no formal leadership that people recognize.

Primary healthcare services and community education are effective only to the extent to which they are accepted in the community. If the practices are embedded into the community with the active involvement of its leaders, sustainable change is possible. For example, after the war in Sierra Leone, young people would not listen to their leaders because they grew up in a war zone, where the normal village structure did not exist. They did not grow up in the traditional system, so a medical system that engages only the local leaders might be ineffective for reaching these young people and persuading them to seek out Western medical care.

I returned to Sierra Leone 20 years after my first

trip, this time with International Medical Corps, who responded to the devastating civil war that erupted in 1991. This assignment was my third with IMC. I worked with them twice in South Sudan, first in 1995 and then again in 1999. It was my first time being back in Sierra Leone since the war broke out.

It was as though a big spoon had stirred up the country. Everyone was displaced. Families, communities—everything was broken up, so the traditional structures for dealing with challenges were completely disoriented.

Like everything else, the initiation to the women's secret society bush had sped up. Now, girls can complete their initiation in two or three days during a school break rather than in two or three months. This means that they are still circumcised, but they miss the camaraderie of the other girls who go through the ceremony with them. And most of all, they do not have the opportunity for a time in which they transform psychologically from girls to women.

We were providing medical care to former child soldiers, children who had been abducted by the rebels and forced into combat or servitude to them. Most had spent their young lives with an armed weapon in their little arms and power and decision-making in the hands of their commander; or they were servants, some of them sexually, to their rebel masters.

Treating their physical ailments was not the challenge—it was teaching them a new way to perceive themselves, with independent life skills and healthier behavior.

We wanted to educate them on personal health and hygiene, but they had no experience learning new behaviors without the threat of a beating looming over them. It was also difficult to help our national health workers teach them in more creative ways than lecture, so we all had to come up with new ways to communicate in this postwar environment.

I lived in Sierra Leone for four years; then, in 2004, I moved to Darfur, Sudan, with International Medical Corps (IMC). I am still here today. After years of moving around, I know there are no "better places," only different ones. At this point in my life, I prefer to build on my local knowledge and further my work rather than to start again in a new place, trying to learn how things are done.

But "settling down" in Darfur is far from settled.

Because of the security situation, we live within the constraints of do's and don'ts. We cannot go anywhere by foot. Just this past February (2009), some international aid workers were kidnapped. The IMC vehicles, with our blue-and-white logo painted on the side, make us an obvious target, so we now have to use rental vehicles. Somehow, we manage to function every day normally. The do's and don'ts become routine, like our 8 p.m. curfew.

I have never been shot at, but in February 2007, one of our teams at one of our sites was attacked in an attempted carjacking. Back at base, I had to communicate with the team and the police to get them back safely. No one was killed, but one woman, a Ministry of Health worker, was shot in the leg. We were on a Medevac flight the next day—the woman who was shot, the expatriate doctor, and I—so that the security situation could be evaluated.

But I am still here. I have left and come back, even under the threat of international kidnappings, to continue my work. When I fly into the airport, I cover my head, particularly on the roads to the compound. I need to make myself less visible on the open roads.

Why am I still doing this?

What my high school yearbook predicted was just the beginning. I cannot pinpoint one specific trigger for wanting to do this work. It's much more insidious than that. They say it gets into your blood and you cannot escape it. After 30 years, I still haven't escaped, but then again, I don't want to. This is the life I chose and every day when I look around, I know how incredibly lucky I am that I have the fundamental liberty to choose.

The Gift of David

~

J. Cloud, RMA

LIVING IN WESTERN KENYA holds many challenges —lack of water, power, food, education, medical staff, and supplies, to name just a few. Amidst this difficult part of the world I met David when he was only a few weeks old, and already he looked like an old man. His story is the same as that of many; it's his gift that's remarkable.

David has three mothers. Two of them saved his life. I'm mom number three. And this is David's story: He was born at just 26 weeks, in a small rural hospital in Kenya; everyone knew that he wasn't going to make it. The nurses would murmur about his delivery in hushed tones, as if David might hear and somehow be made more human.

The awful truth was that he wasn't wanted.

David did not enter the world quietly; he came in wailing. His mother had used a knife to force an abortion.

Mama David delivered her son on the filthy hospital floor. Enraged or horrified—no one knows—she kicked her son across the floor and onto the opposite wall. And still David wailed.

Mama David was bleeding.

Mama David's chart says that the nurses tried to calm her down but that she was insane. She raved. The doctor was called repeatedly, but he didn't come that night. He had no petrol in the car. Mama David died about 30 minutes after she delivered.

Baby David kept breathing. For three days he lay in the incubator, a gift from a very kind donor. The problem was no electricity. And there was no one there to feed him. There was no one to take care of him. No one wanted him, and that's when baby David met his second mom, Sarah.

I have been a nurse since 1999 and have lived in Kenya since 2006 (three years, as I write this). I've specialized in trauma care with bush training. Sarah was a nurse whom I happened to bump into in Kenya. It's funny how it's the people you accidentally meet who become your good friends. I live in the village of Ukwala; Sarah lived in another village, about an hour away, called Siaya. I set up medical clinics for the Siaya hospital with foreign doctors, as well as offered trauma care when it was needed. I was in the hospital a lot during this time, so when I met this little white nurse in a rural hospital, in pretty much the middle of nowhere, we bonded straight away. I met Sarah just before she met David.

Sarah was an American volunteer nurse at the rural hospital. We didn't work together, but we laughed and cried together. Africa is hard; the medical side of Africa is harder. Working in the rural villages with few supplies, little help, and sometimes no clue what to do was the hardest of all. It was enough to make the most seasoned person run away. But Sarah didn't run. She met David; she heard his story, and then he stole her heart. I think that's the day she named him.

David was small, only 1.5 kilograms at birth (a little over three pounds), and by the time Sarah found him he was down to 0.9 kilograms (less than two pounds), but he was still breathing.

I remember Sarah telling me about her "little man." I remember the pride in her voice. Sarah was right. David was a true miracle. So began the day-and-night ordeal of trying to keep little David alive.

I wasn't around for much of this part of David's life. Sarah was everything to him. She kept him alive while she worked at the hospital and took care of her other patients. I would get the occasional phone calls about David, but always I thought that it was only a matter of time before Sarah's heart would be broken. I'd seen babies hold on for a few days, but eventually they died because they knew they weren't wanted. But because of Sarah, David knew he was wanted. That's part of why he lived, but there is still more story for David to tell.

Troubles in Kenya seem to be around every corner. Someone always has something to fight over. It wasn't long, only a couple of months after Sarah and David came together, that Sarah's troubles began. There was a problem with some of the heads of the hospital. As I understood it, one of the witch doctors wasn't happy with Sarah being there and the village was a bit unsettled over some long-dead argument. I never really knew the whole story, but the family she was staying with was actually threatened.

Sarah was upset, but she knew she had to leave. She didn't want to put her home-stay family at risk, and her own parents were concerned over her safety as well. She had to depart Kenya for good; and once again David needed a home.

Sarah asked if I would take him. I was petrified. What was I going to do with a baby that was thriving, but only because of Sarah? What if I was too busy with the clinic, school, and my own kids? I guess I was worried about what would happen to *me* if he came to live with us. I didn't want to get attached to someone so fragile. I told Sarah none of this, only promised that I would do everything I could for him. Everything wasn't going to be enough, but Sarah and I were still so invested in his living that his dying seemed impossible.

David moved in with me and my family and began his life with yet another mom. It wasn't easy. He required 24-hour care. He had to be fed, weighed, and kept healthy. I was continually disinfecting the house, and keeping people with colds away. It was a full-time job.

It became a bit of a routine, but rather quickly my lack of sleep became an issue. All night David would scream and wail. I would hold him, rock him, and sing to him, but nothing would make him settle down.

My days were full of the chaos of family—seven people in two bedrooms. At night, everyone slept but David and me. At first I was angry when he would start wailing at bedtime. I shouted. I cried. I pleaded with him to stop. But he didn't listen; he just screamed. Praying for a miracle seemed easier than praying for him to stop. It was then that I finally gave up, gave in, and asked what I was intended to learn from this experience. I prayed, read my Bible, and prayed some more. Nothing. So, I prayed and prayed until one evening the Lord told me something that blew me out of the water. From then on, I cried every time baby David did.

Little David was grieving. He had lost everything. He was only months old, but he knew he wasn't wanted. He *knew*. He was wounded in his spirit. Once I realized this I was devastated, but from then on he was allowed to cry.

Every night I would rock him and tell him how sorry I was. I, too, had suffered loss, but I'd never truly grieved. I couldn't imagine being tossed aside, kicked, hated, and left to die, and yet baby David knew the agony of such loss. He had nothing else to do but wail.

Another couple of weeks went by and as we rocked all night, I began to understand how truly devastating a wounded spirit can be. I thought of the losses I'd had, of the wounding I'd received. Nothing came even close to what baby David was suffering. I'd never really thought about it, but I guess many of us never truly grieve for our losses. I remember crying when my father died, but did I grieve with every part of me like this baby? I didn't know whether I knew how. But little David didn't have to be taught.

His grief seemed to burn out after about a month. It seemed longer, but I think that was because of the lack of sleep. Then he slept all night one night, and again the next night. I thought my prayers had finally been answered.

David started showing signs that something was seriously wrong when he was about three months old. His eyes started to wander. He couldn't focus or control them. My heart sank the first time I saw it—it meant that there was something wrong with his brain. Something bad was going on. We rushed to the nearest city, then on to yet a bigger one. The CT scan (computed tomography scan, an imaging process that combines special X-ray equipment with sophisticated computers to produce multiple internal images of the body) showed fluid on his brain, and it was building up. He needed a drain, but he was so small that no one in Kenya could perform one, and it would take time to arrange for outside treatment. Time was one thing baby David didn't seem to have.

He started not being awake very much. Early on, I came to the realization that there was nothing we could do. He was too small. At three and a half months, he weighed 3.2 kilograms (about seven pounds). That was it, the fruit of all our efforts: 3.2 kilograms. We had just celebrated his weight the day before his CT. All the strides forward suddenly seemed insignificant. Baby David was dying, and there was nothing that any human could do. I prayed and prayed for baby David's healing. I couldn't understand why he should die, after having lost everything already; he should live to tell about it. He should become a great man.

The first time he stopped breathing was in the middle of the night. I was asleep with him in my arms. I woke up knowing. He didn't sound right. I was frantic. I gave him a few breaths and he kicked awake, wailing like only David could. He was angry with me, but alive and breathing.

I lay in bed after that, afraid to sleep. I prayed he would live, that the Lord would give him back. Then I guess we fell asleep again.

In the morning I knew that the Lord was going to take him home, and it was I that was being selfish. I had to let him go. We went back to the hospital and told the doctors that we wanted a DNR (do not resuscitate) order and pain medications. I wanted David to die at home, surrounded by the love and warmth of our family. He was warm, comfortable, held, and loved. He lived another three days. He never cried again. He didn't scream, either. He smiled. He smiled and watched the rest of the family with interest. His eyes stopped wandering and he watched my face. He looked straight at me when I spoke. At dinnertime the third night, he had been down for a nap when he started to wail. His wailing was so loud that it froze everyone in the house. I thought he was having a bad dream. And then, David was gone.

David had three moms. One was quick to throw him away, while the other two fought to keep him. In the end, baby David won. He survived. He was loved. He grieved his loss. And he died in peace.

I was devastated for a long time. I didn't understand. I didn't want to understand. But then my stepdad sent me an email, and it all made sense.

"I know David is very grateful, as is Jesus, that you are doing what you are doing. So thank Jesus for being able to be a part of David's life, and know that David touched many lives," his email read.

That was it. David was a gift. I am blessed to have known him.

African Odyssey

~

Anna Gersman, RN, BScN

I WAS a naïve white Canadian woman when I followed my South African husband out to Cape Town in
1984, to live and pursue a nursing career. Throughout the
subsequent years of nursing training and work, I was constantly confronted with the laws of separation that created so many powerful barriers in this beautiful country.
I saw firsthand both the hopelessness of poverty and the
privilege of the affluent, which was the reality of South
Africa. I was eager to practice as a nurse, to learn and
experience as much as possible of this strange new world
of nursing and Africa.

The specialty children's hospital where I worked after
graduation was not large, but it was the only center of
its kind in the whole sub-Saharan continent. I wanted to
work with children and was hired to work at a 14-bed

surgical intensive care unit. It was a dumping ground for everything from liver transplants to kwashiorkor and marasmus, the diseases of malnutrition.

I quickly learned to say "I'm sorry for the pain" in three languages in the culturally diverse setting as I gave injections, set up IVs, suctioned, changed dressings, and drew blood on my young patients. I used small sentences and gestures to explain my actions, trying to convey friendliness, calmness, and trust.

Sometimes an African child would scream and shrink away from my white face, from the touch of my white hands. I had to call on my colleagues constantly to translate for me. I learned the power of apology. I apologized for everything—for the pain, the suffering, the grief, the injustice.

All my shortcomings as a nurse and a human being were constantly brought into focus as I nursed my young patients. One weekend, an African in her early teens was brought to the unit. She was severely burned when the shack she was in caught fire. Her burns covered 90 percent of her body. Our goal was to nurse her carefully as she died. She looked out at me from her white-bandaged head. We could not understand each other; I could only convey to her my pity, my comfort, and my deep regret.

It took her mother days to reach the hospital. The patient had come by ambulance, but the mother lived and worked at another location. When the mother finally arrived, I expected her to start crying, screaming, and keening, but she did not. Her calm silence was more frightening. She walked slowly into our mysterious realm, our alternate parallel universe. She waited patiently and respectfully in the doorway and had to be ushered slowly inside. Her frozen footsteps fell silently on the floor in slow motion.

I took her to her daughter, lying in a bed swathed in white bandages, motionless. The mother's head moved from side to side, a slow shaking as if to refocus this vision before her. The daughter's monitor started to race as she recognized her mother. Had her mother come to rescue her, to protect her, to save her? The mother could only stand frozen, helpless at the bedside. We could do little for the girl besides administer massive doses of antibiotics, hydration, and pain medication, as her body slowly shut down.

As a nurse, my heart is broken as I suffer silently with my patients and their families. No tears were shed there at that moment for the pain and life lost. We increased the girl's sedation to calm her, and gave her a dream world to visit. I hoped it would allow her to drift back home with her mother, far from this center of excellence, of medical experts hovering, of machines buzzing and alarms ringing. Maybe home was the valley of a thousand hills where the scent of cooking fires inside little *rondovels* (roundhouses), lingered in the air.

Some days, after my shift, I almost ran to my little blue Volkswagen bug parked beneath the jacaranda tree at the front of the hospital. I could feel the pain and suffering chasing after me as I ran down the stairs and out into the African sunrise or sunset. I inhaled the fresh, clean air and let the hospital doors close behind me, locking down the misery inside. I went home to wash away the smells, to drown out the sounds, to be reborn in the sunlight.

Like any new nurse I yearned to do a good job, to learn the required skills, but I was young; I wanted to have fun, too, and did not want to carry the burdens of this work away with me. On my days off, I escaped into the magnificent landscapes surrounding Cape Town; there were breathtaking vistas of ocean or mountain spreading out in every direction. I felt myself developing confidence as a nurse and a person.

Another day a little brown-skinned toddler lay in a bed with his arm surgically slit open from shoulder to wrist, a fasciotomy to relieve the pressure and restriction to his circulation. He had tried to pick up an injured snake, and the venom had traveled rapidly from the puncture wound on his fat little hand up his arm. The surgeons thought it had to have been an immature snake; if it had been a healthy adult snake, the boy would be dead.

His mother sat on a hard stool at his bedside, her big pregnant belly weighing her down. She did not ask for food or a comfy bed or even a chair. She sat until she was offered some tea or toast. "Thank you," she whispered with a bowed head, hands cupped around the white-china hospital-issue teacup.

We watched and charted the boy's chest rising and falling with a rapid desperation. We watched to see if the poison had stopped moving. Snake venom is cytotoxic, a destroyer of cells. It causes massive swelling and cuts off the victim's circulation.

The emergency room had access to all the snake-bite antidotes: black mamba, boomslang, puff adder, and cobra. In the lunchroom, the African nurses and doctors told stories about scorpions and snake bites. In Africa a backyard was a dangerous place; the houses were pushing farther and farther into the wilderness, and the snakes had nowhere to hide. Construction workers beat the ground with sticks to chase them away as they cleared the ground for new houses.

Yes, I really was in Africa, far, far away from my Canadian roots.

My nursing role was varied. One day I held my breath and steadied my hand as I reached over and plucked the little black leeches, now engorged with blood, off my patient's forehead. I placed them carefully in a plastic container full of muddy brown water at the bedside.

"Good job, Susan," I said as I released my breath. She smiled up at me from under the new forehead the plastic surgeons had created for her.

"Thank you," she whispered in Afrikaans, and closed her eyes.

I looked carefully at the grafted flap to see if the leeches had done the trick of encouraging blood flow from the graft bed into the flap. Susan, and three of her siblings, had been in the back of a little pickup truck that was hit by another car. She was thrown out onto the road, her forehead dragging along the pavement. The implementation of laws regarding seatbelt use, car seats, and restrictions to riding in the back of open vehicles were much looser there. I saw many child victims of terrible preventable accidents. I finished the charting on my ten-year-old patient, pleased that I had hidden my revulsion from her, and turned to the next bed.

While I nursed my patients in the intensive care unit (ICU), a terrible struggle was taking place outside. An international effort to release Nelson Mandela from prison and dismantle apartheid was underway, using economic sanctions. Activists, both black and white, disappeared or were shot in broad daylight. Bold actions occurred in the dying throes of a desperate regime—the collapse of apartheid was coming. People left in the middle of the night for London or Harare.

In the hospital, injustices were apparent too. In my early days, a patient's father asked me, "Is this the white ward?" I just looked at him; I didn't understand the question, and his accent was hard to understand.

I blushed with embarrassment when it dawned on me what he was saying. "I don't know, sir, I'll find out," I said and I stormed off to my colleagues.

They laughed at me and told me how the hospital was once divided strictly into white and non-white sections. Staff and patients were completely segregated. The apartheid laws were slowly being disregarded, and the hospital wards had become racially mixed. The city buses were slowly desegregating, along with the restaurants, beaches, schools, and other places.

One day while chatting with my colleagues, I learned that the pay was different for white, colored, and black nurses. Once again I could only give them a blank, shocked stare.

The colored (mixed race) and black nurses had their own smaller, rowdier tearoom full of boisterous laughter and impromptu comedy. I stood at the door, and a tone of respectful silence descended like a wet blanket. "Hello, sister," they called to me. The registered nurses are called "sisters" following the British medical system. I turned away and went to the quiet, large room reserved for the white nurses. A few colored nurses were in there—no one would dare turn them out. They are serious, hardworking, and overly competent. Apartheid was crumbling; they would soon get equal pay.

Some days I approached the unit with weariness and fear. But as I entered my colleagues called out to me with cheer, eager to hand over to me and keep the cycle of care going. Despite my doubts and fears, I seemed to be pulling my weight; I was part of a team. I was being accepted.

My colleagues liked to put their favorite patients in the bed by the window. One day the patient had a head injury and lay hooked up to a ventilator as we gave medication to reduce brain swelling. I charted her vital signs and tried to soothe her anxious mother, who was keeping watch at her bedside. The child thrashed around wildly for days while her mother kept up a steady whispered conversation of faith and hope. We all waited, observed pupil dilations, and assessed the girl's levels of consciousness.

Her mother seemed to connect into the right level of consciousness. She prayed continuously, as only a mother in that situation can. Gradually the girl improved, her intubation tube was removed, and she was transferred out of our unit.

One day, months later, a tall brown girl stood at the door of the unit. I could have wept when I saw that wild head of long, kinky hair tied up carefully with an elastic. When she was my patient in the bed by the window, I had not seen the huge smile that now lit up the room.

One big brown eye looked around at us all. The other eyelid had some residual paralysis and was to be operated on shortly. Her mother stood beside her, informing us, "This is my Shamima, this is my girl!" The other girl, the one we had nursed, was not this girl standing miraculously before us for all to admire.

How many times did we refill the bed by the window? Another day an African girl lay there fresh from the operating room, where the young French surgical intern had just operated. He came in to see his patient post-op with a nauseated look on his face. The young patient had a ruptured bowel—caused by a bolus of worms. The extracted worms had filled the large steel basin in the operating room and had nearly caused her death. Now she lay quietly in bed with oxygen, and IV lines pumped in antibiotics. Her mother sat day in and day out in the chair beside her, unable to afford the daily trip back to the townships now that she was not working. Townships were designated areas primarily black, outside of the city limits; they were huge squatter camps without electricity and with limited water supplies. Extreme poverty existed in this area with high crime and much political unrest. Because of apartheid black and colored people had to live outside the 'white' city and bus in daily long distances this was part of the terrible injustice.

Patient after patient came and went. We treated thousands of sick children in the unit, and many stories did not end happily. I learned about death and the fathomless grief of parents, siblings, and grandparents. I heard the dull thud of desperate parents clutching one another when the news of their loved one's death reached their ears. I watched them howl and sob, and their tremendous sorrow sent cold shivers down my spine. The mourners clung to small brown hands, frail yellow bodies, and broken black bodies.

As a nurse I learned to attempt to console, to offer a hand, a hug, a shoulder for the tears to flow freely upon. Pitiful goodbyes were regular occurrences for us, as were small bodies being wrapped and taken down to the chapel on the first floor for viewing.

One grieving mother had six pregnancies but no living children. All had died of various diseases in childhood. She was now 40 and had lost her last child. She and her husband sat together at the bedside, heads bowed, defeated.

Somehow in this atmosphere of hopelessness, poverty, and death, I learned the mysterious power of trust and faith. Together with my colleagues at work, I watched on TV as Nelson Mandela regained his freedom. He was only ten miles away when he walked out of Pollsmoor prison after 27 years of incarceration. His motorcade passed close by our hospital. The room was hushed with a shocked reverence for this great leader. A new beginning was taking shape in South Africa.

The colonial boot print had stomped down hard on the dreams, customs, and values of the people of this country. The voices of the black women in particular were silent. I saw the mothers sitting stoically at the bedside of their children, not saying anything. They faded into the background, their strength and determination overlooked and undervalued.

As a nurse I understood their silence, their powerlessness. The mighty strength of our acts of compassion and our nursing skills were universal and basic to human survival, just like these African mothers.

It was in that unit, as barriers and divisions fell, that I formed a strong sense of who I am as a nurse and a person. It was an incredible privilege and honor to work and care for patients at the tip of the African continent. I felt like a true nurse, filled with compassion, kindness, and respect for my patients, and in turn I felt their respect and appreciation for everything I did.

The Small Scheme of Life

~

Mary Catlin, MPH, BSN

As a nurse you can end up taking care of anybody. After a prison riot you stitch up the eyebrows of guards and the ears of convicted bank robbers. You give bed baths to senators and kneel to cut the toenails of rapists. And if you really believe that healthcare is a right, not a privilege, you may end up taking care of both the victims and perpetrators of war.

In 1994 I was working as a public health nurse in a refugee camp for Rwandan refugees, which served the Hutus who had crossed into the eastern Congo and killed about 800,000 of their Tutsi fellow countrymen. At the time it was assumed that perhaps 20,000 Hutu had participated in the genocide, and these were included among the million Hutu refugees. No one really knew. I was there working during the shigellosis, cholera, and meningitis epidemics that were exacting a certain revenge on the Hutus. The first day, I counted 2,000 dead bodies.

This refugee camp, Mugunga, crowded people onto a site on the aptly named Mountains of the Moon as tightly as if all of Seattle had moved their families into plastic pup tents on a few vacant city blocks.

The world here was tilted. Steep slopes bearing banana and papaya trees fell from smoking volcanoes into a huge lake that weeks earlier had been clotted with bodies, and weeks before that had been a water-skiing resort. The first bodies in the waters were Tutsis who had floated from Rwanda after the genocide. Then those disappeared and were replaced by other bodies, Hutus and Congolese who had been stricken by shigella and cholera. Everyone—refugees, genocidists, foreign workers, U.N. forces, and the evil Zairian military in their jaunty red berets—shared, if nothing else, an unsettling concern about the disturbingly active volcano. We all cast an occasional eye on its red glow and ensuing plumes.

We had divided the estimated 300,000 persons in this camp into sections of about 100 households. In my job as the public health coordinator, I walked through each of my sections to check in with my Rwandan staff about the birth and death tolls that we used to see whether the situation was improving or worsening.

To get to Section B, I walked through the narrow spaces that separated the blue plastic sheets that formed shelters. The refugees called these sheetings, which the French aid workers unfailingly corrected to *plastiques*—as if corruption of the French language were the issue most at stake here.

I walked between the sheetings and over to Beane, the head worker in Section B. He handed me his tally paper, on which he tracked the day's events of the 100 families in his section. On the paper were marked the causes of the four deaths: diarrhea, bloody diarrhea, watery diarrhea, and in slanted letters, *Tutsi*.

"Tutsi?" I asked. He took me over to the exposed body of a woman. Usually families or even strangers wrapped bodies in reed mats or in blankets and laid them out on the side of the road for the cemetery workers to pick up in the daily truck run. Usually only feet stuck out the end. The woman was lying with her arms and legs splayed in an X. Around her was the only open space in the entire camp. It looked as though someone had cut her under her arms with a machete and then pulled until her shoulders had dislocated and she bled out. It was a tilted place.

I put her legs together. But the problem—the most immediate problem—was that we needed a blanket to cover her, to give her both some dignity and some ano-nymity, and to carry her out to the road. Usually the work-ers could pick up the ends of the blanket and the feet, or carry someone by the hands and feet, but that was not pos-sible in her case. There was so little one could do to show respect that the public health workers had developed small rituals that came to mean something. No dragging. Lift.

I had few illusions that as a public health nurse I was of value beyond being a distributor of things, a connection to a foreign aid agency with funds, and a keeper of a very few spare blankets.

Oh, I did have illusions. I wanted to keep people alive for a world in which their crimes would be judged by courts of law, not by aid agencies' decisions to give, or withhold, food, water, and medical care. And I tried to keep my organization's aid from being used for direct military assistance. Both efforts were no doubt futile and naïve. But focusing on the small scheme, I felt that this woman had earned her blanket. I got one to wrap her in and gave it to Beane.

I made my way to the headquarters tent at the edge of camp to let the camp head know that a woman had just been murdered, but I never got the chance. Pierre, the French Camp coordinator, stood listening to the walkie-talkie at his ear. He looked unhappy.

"There is a Tutsi woman who has taken refuge in the clinic compound saying she will be killed, and a mob outside wants her to be turned over to them." He knew that I went in and out of the clinic all morning with stretchers as the Community Health Workers (CHW) identified people in the sections who needed care, and I approved referrals.

"I could go transport a patient, and see what's up," I said. He agreed. I got help and loaded up someone we had found collapsed alongside the road.

The clinic was partway up the hill, conducted in two old army tents surrounded by a waist-high red rock wall. The wall of hand-placed rocks marked the border between the milling crowd on the outside and the clinic space, where 100 patients lined up inside.

The wall had been built stone by stone by a small group of young men, who were unfailingly cheerful and hard-working. I often took them my high-energy biscuits at lunch, which I handed over with a small prayer that they had not been directly involved in the massacre of hundreds of thousands of their countrymen. When they dug the latrine in the volcanic rock it took three weeks with sledgehammers, and then they used an imported jackhammer to get six feet deeper in the hard rock. The irony was that if they were murderers, all I could do was withhold biscuits, and ask them *not* to do the hard-labor building of a latrine.

The compound's rock wall had a gap big enough for two cars to enter and was guarded by a graying man, who had tied from one edge of the gap to the other a red string, which he moved majestically to allow the trucks to enter and depart. As I came up the hill, trying to wedge the crowds open for the stretcher, thousands of people were on the road surrounding the clinic but no one had yet crossed the line marked by the red string.

One or two young men were coaching the crowd yelling in Kinyarwandan, "Give us the Tutsi or else!" However, they paid the stretcher no attention and let us duck under the string and enter the clinic compound.

The expatriates were knotted in between the two tents. Louis Braille, at that time a physician in his 60s, had immediately gotten the Tutsi woman out of sight. I peeked at her as she sat on the mats in one of the tents. She was in her 30s and dressed, quite remarkably, in Levis. She was breastfeeding a baby and soothing a four-year-old at her side. My Hutu workers, who had returned for lunch break, were sitting a little away from her, but they had at least shared their high-energy biscuits and some water with her.

I asked Louis what I should tell headquarters. He thought. "Well, if we expats leave, they'll get her sooner..." And he resumed examining a gray-haired woman with flat breasts like triangular pockets. She, like me, was distracted by the increasing volume and agitation of the crowd. Louis asked her patiently about her cough and she responded nervously, "*Commez? Commez?*" (Kinyarwanda-French slang similar to "Come again?" or "What?"). The other patients in line had quietly picked up their red-stitched blankets and left the compound. I called the health workers, Philipe, Claude, and Anton, to accompany me back out into camp. We ducked under the red string and left.

Back at headquarters, I updated Pierre and he, in turn, informed me that the United Nations had contacted a Hutu officer at Lac Vert. The officer was coming over to negotiate. It was understood that the more aid agencies that pulled out, the less there was for the Hutu military to steal. That we needed the Hutu military to settle this was also an indication of the level of the military's control over the refugees.

Pierre sent me back up the hill to tell the clinic staff to try to hold on. I found a kid with a pus-filled leg in the crowd and told him we'd take him for a ride. In front of the clinic, a young lead agitator in the crowd of thousands had now grabbed a terrified-looking man by the collar of his red shirt, someone who moments before had been a spectator yelling for blood. He held the man in a choke-hold, with others restraining his arms, and said, "Give us the Tutsi or we will kill him." The small red string still held the crowd back by a repellant force, and by obscure courtesy the crowd still parted to let us through. But they were closer, now pushing against the string. Several people had shown up with torches that they held high to avoid igniting the dense crowd. Were they going to light our tents on fire? Burn the Tutsi woman alive?

Louis turned to me and said matter-of-factly, "We should get her kids to the orphanage now." He meant, "so they won't be killed too." So I radioed for my community health workers, took the stretcher, and went into the tent with the Tutsi woman.

I held out my arms to the woman. What was the French to explain that she should give me her children in case we might not be able to save her? She immediately understood and wordlessly handed over her small child, doing absolutely nothing to upset the child. Her immediate selfless gesture, with her own life at risk, was an epiphany for me of what courage is, of what mothers sacrifice for their children. I have never forgotten the moment. She gestured that she would keep the baby. I nodded, not trusting my voice. I went into the other tent, got three Hutu kids to use as camouflage, and put all four small kids on the cot under the blanket, covering the little Tutsi lest his better clothes give him away.

Walking into an enraged crowd of Hutus with machetes while carrying a Tutsi is one of those harrowing moments of life, like stepping out of an airplane at 10,000 feet. But as we had done all day, we walked out with the stretcher as if we were transferring patients to the malnutrition tent, the hospital, or in this case the orphanage. The crowd parted enough to let us through. I didn't look back as I headed toward the top of the hill.

We climbed steadily, past the huge pit that served as the cemetery. It sometimes looked like a field of mushrooms when people were buried too shallowly and the postmortem gases pushed swollen toes up through the pumice.

We walked past the latrine project, past the World Food Program food storage, up to the top of the orphanage. The camp thinned out here; the rocks were too craggy to sleep on, and the seeping volcanic gases sometimes killed those who slept in the deeper crevices. My teeny Tutsi was oblivious, singing to himself.

This orphanage at the top of the hill was run by the Irish and helped sort out some of the 11,000 orphans. I grabbed the completely sensible, absolutely practical, Irish coordinator by the arm and took her to the edge of the compound to speak in private.

"One kid in intake's a Tutsi. We've got to get him out of here," I told her,

"Jesus Mary Mother of God," she said.

I asked for her car and about eight orphans so we

could drive through camp as if we were going to the next orphanage over a few kilometers away. I told her I didn't actually want to leave him until I heard whether his mother was dead.

She looked down and switched her radio over to the security channel. Without discussion, she called up her Rwandan driver, Dr. Rayon, explained that I needed transport, and then selected a group of unaccompanied minors of about the same age that could be transferred. She helped undress the Tutsi of his fancy clean suit with small ducks. He was quite happy to be as naked as his peers, who were quieter and world-weary. We loaded nine small children into the car. Unfortunately, the only unmined road out of camp went directly back in front of the clinic through the mob.

I asked the driver to go to the nearest orphanage. We drove out the gate and the car slipped into the stream of the crowd, able to go only as fast as they walked. Three small kids immediately jumped on the bumper for a free ride. Occasionally the crowd would rock the car to give us a small menacing thrill, but we progressed on, slowly, slowly, until finally the road went directly past the mob at the clinic—now with the young man in the red shirt up on the rock wall with a machete held to his throat, the crowd yelling in rhythmic chants, the local refugee staff apparently gone from the compound, only the expatriates in sight by the back of the tent. No sign of the colonel.

The driver regarded me quizzically for a moment when he saw my green truck in the clinic compound, as this meant I really didn't need his services. He rolled up his window the remaining inches. "For the air conditioning," he said with a smile. He had none. He leaned over to lock the doors that I had surreptitiously already locked. We slipped past, through the middle of the crowd, who rocked the car a few times but were still focused on the clinic.

Thirty minutes later we had gone six kilometers and were out of camp onto an open road. I started to breathe again. The driver stopped and radioed base to come get me. When headquarters' car arrived, I asked the first driver to take the other kids to the orphanage and let him know that I would take this one. Again he looked at me. He was a Hutu, and I didn't know what he knew, or who he knew, or whether he'd tell if he did know. But he said "Okay," and stuck his arms out in front of him. They were shaking all the way up to his shoulders. I took his hand not to shake it but to still it.

"Where I come from in Seattle we'd accuse you of too much coffee," I tried to joke.

"Where I come from…" he said, and his voice caught.

I rode back to my home compound in Goma. The little Tutsi in my lap pulled at my buttons and flirted with gentle brown eyes. He was very soft to hold onto as I awaited instructions on what to do next. I fed him bananas and showed him the green African forest parrots that the Indian landlord owner had left there.

I tried to imagine what was happening in camp and feared for everyone in the clinic compound. Finally, after four nerve-wracking hours, the radio crackled and headquarters asked me to come into the Goma office. I showed my papers, signed the guest book, and walked up the marble stairs of the bank that was now occupied by the United Nations offices. I was ushered into a back office, where to my amazement, I saw the child's mother having tea with the head of the agency.

"You're alive," I said.

"Yes," she answered.

I kissed my little friend and handed him over. She shifted her baby in her arms and restored her second child to her lap so nonchalantly that it completely unnerved me. It was as if nothing had happened.

I had expected both of us to be killed. I had expected to hear that my co-workers were killed. I didn't get it. I guess I was expecting a thank you. "Do you..." I began. "Do you have the least idea why I took your child? Do you know how close you were to being murdered?"

"Yes," she said in a sharp hiss that made it clear that things were not over for her, and if I expected thanks for stepping up one time, while she and others risked their lives continuously and would need to for the foreseeable future... She made me feel that this eruption of sentimentality was a *muzungu* (a white-skinned person) luxury from another world.

Get over it; it is no big deal.

Access to camp services closed for a few days, despite the negotiations with the colonel. The man in the red shirt was beaten up but lived. The other clinic workers were escorted out of camp. Dutch commandos appeared from nowhere, sent by The Office of the United Nations High Commissioner for Refugees, who, to their credit, managed to get the mom and her children out of the Congo and back into Rwanda.

Weeks later we heard that she was not a Tutsi.

Burst Wide Open

~

Heather Starshine McLeod, MSN, ARNP

HORTON FARM CAMP for Internally Displaced Persons, Liberia, West Africa: I am now imprinted with a fear, hatred, and dread of Horton Farm, simply because the people are so, so sick here, and our two worst days, so far, have been here. This week we saw 322 people in one day, a new high for us, in a clinic day that defies description. Everyone is spiking a temp—temps of 104, 105°F. *How far up does a digital thermometer go?* And we are trying madly to crush Tylenol and figure out the right doses and get it into these little infants that have been seizing with these high temps in the night. I see an 11-year-old with a temp of 104°F—and the translator is yelling at her because she is not answering my questions. Her brain is on fire—how can one expect her to talk straight!

In a day in which everything has gone wrong, we somehow forgot to load up our chairs in the morning and so we are sitting on wooden planks, or on tops of tables, and my back is killing me. It is, as always, too hot to think. Midway through the day, when I go to drink water in a mad attempt to avoid my daily dehydration headache, I find that ants have crawled inside my water bottle. There is no other clean water for miles. In fact, Horton Farm is our one camp that has had trouble getting any water at all on some days, and I can't bear to ask anyone if they might have some to spare.

I am stupid with exhaustion by the time we usually are wrapping up, unable to think anymore, and yet when I get up to look out at the line of waiting patients, I find that it looks just as long as it did in the morning. As more time goes by, more people know that we come to certain camps on certain days, and so they walk for hours out of the bush to come to be examined, even if they are not from the camps themselves. All of our camps are within the United Nations "bubble"—the name given to the area controlled by U.N. forces, and therefore considered relatively safe. As the security condition in the country becomes more and more stable and this bubble expands, people from the bush also feel safe enough to venture out to visit one of our camps, whereas before, they might be have been wary of leaving their homes. As a result, our patient numbers are increasing and I don't see how we can sustain them with this level of staff, but that is not my problem to solve.

At any rate, by the time we have staggered our way through everybody, we are two to three hours late and nobody has eaten. And of course, this day of all days, someone has forgotten to put in our lunch supplies and all we have is plain bread. I am so, so tired. And this after a day of having my own high fever and sickness. I am so woozy and weak that I literally cannot see straight and keep having to blink my eyes to focus. And so I make an executive decision to drink my water, ants and all. Well, none of the ants actually go down my throat, of course I see to that, but there is no way to mentally trick yourself into forgetting that little dirty critters have been swimming around in your drink!

We finally pull away at the end of the day with three itty-bitty infants to transport, all less than five months old and all so sick that I am afraid they might die in the car on the way back. One of them is from somewhere just past Horton Farm, and the mother wants us to swing by her house to pick up some of her clothes before heading to the hospital. She says it is not far, but in truth it is at least an extra hour out of our way, and we go careening out a little, dinky dirt road with our antenna smashing into the overhanging trees, pigs lying in puddles, our three little sick ones being jounced around in the back.

We pull up to this little village out in the middle of nowhere—maybe ten or so huts in a cluster, with outside walls decorated with paint imprints made in the shapes of leaves and of something that looks like it must have been a chicken foot ... quite pretty, actually. Truth be told, this sleepy little clump of homes looks sort of nice ... very primitive, to be sure, but a happy-looking community. Little kids (and in fact, the whole village) come running to the car, and we sit and wait while the mother grabs her things and everyone thanks us for carrying the child. One can see, being in this place, why the people in the camps want so badly to go home to their own villages, which, unlike this one, are often still unsafe because they are outside the U.N. bubble. This life is still hard, but it feels much more nurturing than the camps with their unending rows of huts and crowding.

Back on the road, we drive toward home with only one of the infants crying a sick little occasional squawk. I take her squawk as a good sign, because perhaps this kid is fighting. She is a three-month-old with eyes yellow as butter, totally jaundiced and with a rock-hard belly and high temp. Malaria with hepatic involvement? Hepatitis, maybe? Passed from the mom at birth? It could be yellow fever, since we've heard reports of outbreaks here, but apparently once people with yellow fever get jaundiced they are usually hemorrhaging, and this little kid isn't bleeding as far as I can tell.

Our second kidlet is a two-month-old cutie with a pretty clear case of malaria. He has a fever of 104°F, and is so anemic that his little palms and soles look white. He has been sick for only a few days, according to his mom, but he does not look good and he won't suck, although he chokes down the Tylenol in water that we pour into his tiny mouth. The third little one is five

months old, temp of 103.7°F, with diarrhea and vomit-
ing. I go automatically to feel her fontanel (the "soft
spot" on the top of the head), expecting it to feel sunken
with dehydration, expecting to simply give antimalarial
medicine and Tylenol and loads of oral rehydration salts,
and likely some antibiotics, since the mom says there is
blood in the diarrhea. And instead of the classic inden-
tation near the front of her skull, I find an outpushing,
bulbous anterior fontanel—shit... Something else is
going on, something to increase the intracranial pressure
—encephalitis, meningitis? I don't know! And so she is in
the car with us now as well.

How can I say how I feel at the end of this day? Totally
spent, worn, damaged, and empty. With every challenge
that happens here, I understand more—and then immediately less. Half of the time I am me, just like always, and
then half of the time I don't know who I am. Why I am
here and why I am alone and why I am a nurse and why
I am not a Liberian IDP or an Iranian opium-grower or a
Swiss watchmaker or a Cambodian farmer. Or a French
acrobat for the Cirque du Soleil—which is what I really
want to be, especially at that moment—spinning around
in the air with a costume of chiffon and feathers and little
spiral, fuzzy wires springing from a beautiful, outrageous,
sparkling mask, me bouncing in perfect symmetry with
other such beings, heart beating strongly with music cas-
cading around me and with no fear of falling.

And yet ... I am not this.

We drop off our little patients and their caretakers, and

I do my rounds at the hospital in a fog, then go home to compile stats for the day—how many patients seen, how much diarrheal illness, what meds were given. My head swims with faces and names, and some of my own stats from the day don't even look familiar to me at all. And then pumpkin soup for dinner, our absolute favorite, and off to bed in my little mosquito-netted world, so hot and sweaty that rest is fitful as always, and I dream endlessly of having countless tasks that I am somehow never able to complete, always leaving something out or doing something wrong or forgetting what I was doing in the first place.

The next day's camp is better, not as relentless as Horton Farm, but still exhausting and emotional. When we return to the compound at the end of the day, I head to the hospital dutifully to do my rounds. But the minute I walk in, I can tell by the nurses' expressions that something is wrong. Simply put, our little malaria boy, with the pale, pale palms and soles, is dead. His hemoglobin was 4.5, for goodness sake—4.5, when normal for him would be about 12! They transfused blood and gave him IV quinine for malaria as soon as we brought him in, and he lived through the night, but he just didn't have the physical resources to make it. Just couldn't rebound from the place he had been thrust by some stupid parasite in some stupid mosquito.

There is the mom, standing in front of me, and I think, my God, why did I not ask someone what the culturally appropriate response to death is here? Because although there is no "right" thing to say in this situation to anyone, anywhere, I suppose in my own country I could convey my caring and love in some fashion. But here, I don't know how. Should I touch her? Place a hand on an arm? Console her? Should I say something about God? Most people are so very Christian here, but then again, some are Muslim, and people from the bush follow African traditional religions, and I don't know this woman at all—what she believes, what she could possibly be feeling. And, oh, God, she has lost her child!

Yet she is stoic, standing there in front of me without a word, and I don't know whether to be stoic too, or to just break down and fall to the ground and cry, which is what I want to do.

And now, of course, she wants to take the body home with her, but she is the one that lives in the little village, far out on the dirt road, out past our camps, at least a three-hour drive away. And it will be dark soon. And we can put her in a taxi, but no one else will get in the taxi with a dead baby, and the taxi drivers demand all sorts of money to carry a single person. They usually pack about 20 into a little sedan. And a taxi can't make it down the dirt road anyway, so if she goes now, she will be walking, alone, in the dark, along a dirt road, with her dead baby in a cardboard box, and this is quite simply just too awful to comprehend.

But if she stays we lose time, even if we take her to a taxi first thing in the morning. The morgue is not chilled, because the electricity is so intermittent. We can't stand to waste precious time.

And I can't make this make any sense and I want to go home and I want my mommy and I want to click my heels, but how can I be so selfishly thinking about how scared I am when this woman has lost her child?

There is no good option here. How could there ever, ever in a million years, be a good option here? And so we settle on the best plan we can think of, with Peter agreeing to come the next morning, even though it is Saturday and supposed to be our day off, to drive us to the Red Light market district, where we hope to find a car that will agree to carry the woman home.

And so in the glaring heat of the next morning we drive, Peter and I and the mother. As soon as she sees the cardboard box carrying her son loaded up into the back of the vehicle, she breaks down, and now she sits, sobbing, crammed next to me in the car.

She is turned away from me, and all I can do is to try to keep breathing as I stare at a little pink barrette in her hair, old and dirty, and gilded with silly gold lining. And I wonder where she got it, and I don't know why I wonder such a stupid, ridiculous, inconsequential thing at a time like this.

We drive, and outside the world just keeps going as if all is normal, in spite of our journey, in spite of this woman's pain. All the bustle and noise and dirt of the market is screaming in on us, all mundane and normal and fine—but all so totally, brutally, nonsensically inappropriate. I would like to roll up the windows to keep out the sound, but we have to keep the windows down in the vehicle because we don't want the woman to have to smell her baby in its cardboard box.

And so we finally reach the Red Light market area like this, where we pay 20 American dollars for a taxi to take the woman home. And we have to bargain for it. We actually have to sit and bargain with the driver for this awful, awful thing. Peter negotiates the price of taxi fare while the woman sits beside me and I hold my hand on her back, between her shoulder blades, and I try to send every bit of love and strength I can find down through my arm and my hand and my fingers, not knowing if my touch is offending her, but just knowing that it is all I can think of to do.

As we wait for the bargaining to conclude, I buy her a loaf of bread and something pudding-like in texture that comes in a plastic bag, because she has not eaten and I don't know how to help her any more than this. And then she drives away, off into her life. Just like that, so alone and small in the front seat of that taxi, with the cardboard box in the hatchback trunk.

Peter and I drive home, in silence, behind a U.N. tank, with the rear gunner sitting stolidly with the huge tank gun pointed straight at us. I want him to move it away from us, point it up, or sideways or something. I am sure the safety must be on, but what if it isn't and the tank hits a pothole and it accidentally fires? I know this is ridiculously improbable, and I'm sure it is not even loaded, but with the horror of that morning I feel so small and afraid, and now that thing is pointed at me, and I don't like it one bit.

On the way back we pass Benson Hospital, where we dropped our other two kids on Thursday, and although I am terrified of what I will find, I ask Peter to stop so I can check on them. Miraculously, they are both still alive, one with malaria and hepatitis and one with meningitis, but both awake and looking at me from dirty beds with torn, old sheets.

And so, what of me? I am overwhelmed. So past "whelmed." Maybe if I knew where whelmed was, I would crawl back there on my hands and knees and lay my face on the cool, smooth surface of the relative calm of whelmed. In many ways I knew it would be like this, but I don't think it is possible to viscerally feel the depth of this challenge without actually being inside it. The strength that it is taking me to work this hard and to keep myself intact emotionally is a strength that is new to me, one that I didn't know I had. And yet even with all of this chaos and pain, there are also so many moments here when I am just simply fine. I cook an egg for breakfast; read my book on the porch; shop for *lapas*, brightly colored, multi-patterned pieces of cloth, in the market; write email. I brush my teeth at night, and I take my vitamins, and I clean my contacts, and my laundry gets done. I sit and laugh with the people I have met here, people who are seeing all this too, who care about this the way I care about this.

And so, I am strangely okay. How can I explain this? Before dinner tonight, I clear the table and chairs out of a side room in the guest house, and in front of a window looking out on the ocean I place my yoga mat. The window has a filmy curtain of white, see-through, silky material, and it blows softly against my face with the breeze as I move. I haven't done yoga since I've been here. I did try once, but it was too darn hot and I had no energy for it. But now I force myself anyway, with the sweat literally streaming off me, and at one point I have to stop because I am sobbing and I have to hug my knees close to my chest and wait awhile.

I am burst wide open, and still I can tell that I am only scratching the surface of myself. This is what I needed, what I wanted, what I knew I had to chase down when I planned this trip—this pasting of eyes wide open, opening of my heart completely to something so vastly outside of myself, in order to somehow challenge myself in ways that I still don't understand fully.

I want to care for the Liberian people, to witness their lives, to respect their pain. I want to step out of the denial that living in the United States affords me and use my nursing skills to give something back. I can only hope that my presence here offers something of value to these people who have been through so much, because I can already tell that what I am gaining here is valuable beyond words.

PART THREE

Finding Humor

In the Doghouse

~

Fiona MacLeod, BSN

In July of 2008, looking for a bit of adventure, culture, and travel, I left my comfortable research job in Vancouver, British Columbia, and set off to the Middle East. I had accepted a one-year contract working on a ward at a large research hospital in Saudi Arabia. Little did I know at that time that these 12 months were to be the most significant learning experience of my entire life to date, culturally, professionally, and personally.

One of the most significant things I have learned is just how powerful language can be. Making the effort to acquire and use even a limited vocabulary of the local language can create bonds and help to seal off deeply running cultural fissures.

Often, my narrow berth of the Arabic language limits me to using words that I know aren't exactly right in a particular context; however, in most situations, the point usually gets across, and my faltering attempts are generally met with encouragement and endearment. My efforts also provide much-needed comedic relief for both the patient and myself within the sober hospital environment.

Every day I am adding to the list of words that I keep in my pocket, and every night I try to practice each one and commit it to memory. I am proud to say that I can now ask Arabic-speaking patients whether they have moved their bowels today, yesterday, or the day before yesterday; whether they have had any diarrhea; whether they are constipated, and whether they would like any medication to assist in whatever dysfunctional bowel pattern they may be experiencing. Unfortunately, this wealth of knowledge does not transfer well to communication with the general public, such as at shopping malls or with cab drivers.

I should also make clear that at the beginning, while I could get a basic point across, I generally spoke either in very short sentences with devastatingly poor grammar or in single words punctuated with animated gesticulations to get my point across. The latter method was not always well received before I learned all my bowel-related Arabic.

My first language blunder happened in the first week on my new ward. First, a bit of background: Though the holy Qur'an emphasizes kindness to all animals, dogs are considered "dirty" in Islam. Muslims do not keep dogs as pets in Saudi, and generally the only place one can see a dog is in the desert, is with a fleeting glimpse of a wild *saluki*. Touching a dog voids *wudu,* the ritualistic washing of one's self with water prior to each of the five daily *salas* (prayers).

One of my first proud new words was *gelb,* which means "heart." The "g" sound in Arabic is quite soft, and can almost be mistaken for a "k." On one particular day, I was happily doing my morning assessments in my patients' rooms. When it came time to use my newly acquired vocabulary, I would lift my eyebrows, point at the patient's chest, and say "*kelb?*" as in "Can I listen to your heart?" By the third patient, I could not shake the feeling that I was getting a little bit of hostility, although I told myself that it was a cultural thing that I was no doubt misinterpreting.

It wasn't until later on that day, when I was practicing my Arabic with one of my Lebanese co-workers, that I realized my embarrassing blunder. Apparently, I had been pronouncing my "g" sound too softly, and it was coming out as a fairly audible "k." While *gelb* means "heart," unfortunately *kelb* means "dog." In case there was any doubt as to whom I was referring when I uttered the insult, I must remind you that I pointed at my patients' chests while saying it. As an aside, I also found out later that single-finger pointing at someone in any capacity in the Muslim culture is also insulting. Oh, dear—strike two.

My Arabic has come a long way since this first incident, though not without additional and equally amusing blunders. Though I am proud to say that I have developed a fairly good "working knowledge" of the language, I am also aware that in certain situations it is not appropriate to have any ambiguity around what is being said. In some instances, the necessary explanation or command of the language goes far beyond my capability.

A very important lesson I have learned is that sometimes, just staying completely silent while doing your job quickly and expertly speaks louder and more articulately than the most intelligent and thought-provoking exchange in *any* language. In keeping with this, I would also like to share a more recent experience with language.

One of my patients was scheduled for a bone marrow biopsy. If you have ever received, observed, or assisted with a bone marrow biopsy, you know well that "barbaric" is a gross understatement in describing the procedure. The patient lies in a semi-prone position while the doctor drives a needle, roughly the width of a chopstick and the length of your hand, from the wrist to the tip of your baby finger, through layers of dermis and muscle, and into the bony pelvis. The intention is to collect a corkscrew-like sample of bone marrow to analyze for blood cancer.

I say "intention" because often it takes more than one trip of boring the needle through the fleshy tunnel and retracting it to check whether the sample attempt was successful. This procedure is done under a local anesthetic, and a needle as long as your middle finger filled with Xylocaine is driven into the flesh and alternately eased forward and backward to ensure that an adequately wide area has been numbed. The patient gets some pre-medication for pain and anxiety, but I liken this to offering someone a Tylenol and a lavender-oil neck massage before a bilateral leg amputation.

This particular patient had a history of chronic pain and depression, and she was particularly anxious and teary prior to, and during, the procedure. I pulled up a chair beside her bed and held both her hands as I spoke in my best soothing voice, and tried desperately to pass on strength and will to the distraught woman. The woman cried out in pain and clamped my hands in a diaphoretic vise-grip as the needle drove into the back of her pelvis.

The doctor who was performing the procedure is an incredibly intelligent man, meticulously conscious of minute details "behind the scenes." Unfortunately, however, his bedside manner would no doubt cause Florence Nightingale to have a serious nervous meltdown. He is not a native Arabic speaker, but he seemed to truly believe that knowing how to say "Is there pain here?" and "There is not pain; what is the problem?" in Arabic was an acceptable range of vernacular to competently perform this procedure.

As these questions were delivered in his signature manner with a harsh, accusatory "Huh?" after every question, I felt my jaw clench tighter and tighter as the patient's cries grew louder. My "Western-style" temper erupted violently over the edges of the gender-repressed container into which I had packed it, for the time being, in order to assimilate into my new culture.

His third "There is not pain; what is the problem? Huh?" was cut short by my urgent, even statement, which surprised even me as it quietly but forcefully escaped my lips.

"With all due respect, doctor, I think the crying and yelling is fairly indicative of the pain, and the problem is that she has an eight-inch needle the size of a pencil stuck into her pelvis. Can we just get this over with as quickly as possible, please?"

The room was suddenly silent except for the whimpered Qur'an verses escaping the pursed lips of the young woman. You could cut the tension with surgery shears. I met the doctor's patronizing stare calmly and firmly, despite the creeping fingers of crimson that slowly made their way up my neck and prickled my ears.

Just when I was certain that the doctor was going to stalk out of the room, leaving the biopsy needle protruding out of the patient's pelvis like a Saudi oil rig, he broke the gaze, muttering something about protocol. The remainder of the procedure was slightly tense, but thankfully quick, quiet, and relatively uneventful.

Experiences like this one taught me that gaining a handle on the local language is essential but is not enough. It is just as important—even a professional responsibility—to know our limitations, use sound judgment, and be honest about the range of our abilities both to ourselves and with others.

Don't Get Too Fond
of the Pig

~

Louise M. Robinson, RN

Wʜᴇɴ ᴊᴏʜɴ ꜰ. ᴋᴇɴɴᴇᴅʏ created the Peace
Corps in 1961 he also created my dream, but for 25 years
my dream took a backseat to raising a daughter, going to
college, and bringing home the bacon. My dream became
reality when I earned my nursing degree at the age of 45,
joined the Peace Corps, and was assigned to Guatemala.

All volunteers are sent to a training center for three
months to learn about their host country, its habits and
customs, and definitely the language. We had all expected
to be thrown immediately into the wilds of this mountainous country. Instead, our training center was in Antigua,
a lovely little city in the mountains of Guatemala—very
much a wealthy tourist area, with lovely homes and shops.

We each lived with a host family and went to "school" every day. The training center had many different programs, including healthcare, agriculture, and animal husbandry.

The very charming sow who was part of the agriculture program became a close friend. She was about my age (in pig years), and she listened patiently to my comments and complaints while I scratched her bristly back with a stick. She would come at the sound of my voice and swoon onto my side as soon as I started scratching. Then she disappeared—one day before the training center graduation barbeque. I wrote a poem in her honor:

Twinkle

Twinkle, twinkle, little pig,
Looking at you made me sick.
From the depths of yonder dump,
You had risen from your rump.

I recall when I first saw you,
You were covered in slime and goo.
Garbage hanging from your hips,
Rotten carrots in your lips.

How was I to know that day,
To you, my piggy, I would say,
"Come and join me where I sit,
I enjoy your sparkling wit."

How long I'd been at my site,
Struggling with all my might,
Trying to speak another tongue,
Sometimes feeling I'd come unstrung.

Oh, I wished there was a *gringo*,
Someone else who knew my lingo.
Someone with whom I could converse,
To make life better, not worse.

Alas, there was no English spoken,
There I was, my spirit broken.
I started talking to myself,
Then to the roaches on the shelf.

And here is where this strange plot thickens,
I started talking to the chickens.
I spoke my thoughts, my hopes, my dreams,
I'd really lost my mind, it seems.

And then I saw your piggy eyes,
Looking at me … Oh, so wise.
Somehow you knew I had no buddy,
You came to chat, a little muddy.

We talked and talked, it was such fun,
I felt my life had just begun.
We joked and laughed, my sides were achin',
I vowed to you I hated bacon.

Then came the day we had to part.
I swear to you it broke my heart.
They slaughtered you against my wishes,
But, oh, my friend, you were delicious!

Once training was completed, volunteers were assigned a site where they worked, ate, lived, and breathed as the locals did. My site assignment was the tiny village of Oratorio. There I was to find somewhere to live while climbing mountains and fording rivers in my quest to bring healthcare to the local residents.

Once established in Oratorio, I rented a one-room domicile next to my landlady's pigs and chickens. However, I soon discovered there was already a small health center right there in the village where the people for miles around would bring their health needs.

In my frustration at not being able to accomplish much, and in my loneliness, I turned to my landlady's pig for companionship. However, the pig died shortly after eating some of my leftover stew. Alone, again.

I had discussed the situation in Oratorio with my supervisor, and we decided I would be of more use somewhere else. I would stay in Oratorio until another site was found. Most volunteers return to Peace Corps headquarters in the capital, Guatemala City, once a month or so to get mail and information handouts and to visit with other volunteers.

In my case, the trip involved a walk of several miles to get the local "chicken bus" into the capital, then another walk of several miles, through some questionable neighborhoods, to Peace Corps headquarters. The "chicken bus" was an adventure in itself. Passengers were usually accompanied by their entire family, a goat or two, baskets of chickens and other provisions, and sometimes furniture. The bus seldom came to a complete stop, but everyone was most congenial and cheerfully helped me get on and off while it was still moving.

One Sunday another volunteer, Connie, invited me to the grand opening ceremony of a refuge for street children run by a Catholic organization. She introduced me to Padre Miguel, who would be running the place. I was rattling away to him in my fractured Spanish when he smiled gently and said, "I speak English." Father Michael was from Connecticut.

I asked him if he'd like me to come in on weekends and work in the clinic they were setting up for the children. He thanked me profusely. It was always difficult to get anyone to work on weekends. I would assist the male nurse on duty, if there was one, being careful not to presume to know more than he. If there was no other nurse on duty, it was just me and the kids.

I loved the work.

The street kids were starved for affection, and just being spoken to, or touched, was enough to make their week memorable. First they were bathed and deloused. Then they came to the clinic for hugs and whatever medical treatment was needed—vaccinations; treatment for worms, cuts, and bruises.

Father Michael asked me to take pictures of the kids in the street and at the refuge for the fund-raising brochure. He always escorted me when I went out at night to get photos of the children sleeping in doorways and gutters and under cardboard boxes. There were so many of these children. The parents, who were incredibly poor and had many more children than they could feed, would gather the five or ten oldest and bring them to Guatemala City and leave them on the street, hoping they would somehow survive.

The children were quickly gathered in by the other street kids and shown the ropes. They existed by begging and stealing. There were mostly boys on the streets because the girls usually survived by going into prostitution, no matter how young they were.

Another large part of their existence was "huffing"—spraying paint into paper bags and inhaling the fumes. One way to escape the horror of their lives was to be unconscious.

They came to the refuge for food and a safe place to sleep. We fed them, clothed them, and saw to their medical needs. One of the boys brought in his five-year-old brother. The older boy told me his brother said that his legs hurt. I took him on my lap and held him and talked to him until his pain went away.

Father Michael got the five-year-old and his brother to Casa Alianza, the orphanage in Antigua. I visited there when I was in training. It's a beautiful old hacienda where they take very good care of the children and see that they go to school.

A benefactor in the States sent several large boxes of shoes to the refuge. They were all high-top basketball-type shoes, blue with orange laces and trim. The children all knew me by then, and whenever they saw me in Guatemala City I was greeted by screams of *"Abuelita! Abuelita!"* I felt honored to be addressed as "Little Grandmother" by a multitude of filthy urchins—all wearing blue-and-orange shoes.

Along with Father Michael, I was invited to attend the dedication of a new group home in Guatemala City, with all the proper fanfare and the presence of the governor, ambassador, and other officials. My social life certainly had highs and lows.

Eventually I worked almost every week at the clinic in the refuge. My heart just wasn't in Oratorio. The two male nurses who worked at the clinic were typical Latin macho types and demanded the utmost respect from the kids. I got hugs.

The refuge got a donation of some dental equipment and medicines for our clinic, and a dentist from Houston came down to set it up and work on the kids' teeth. I volunteered to help, and soon I was a semi-fledged dental assistant. Most of the children had good teeth and few cavities, in spite of limited oral hygiene. The dentist thought it might be because of the water, or genetics, or any number of reasons.

Father Michael asked me if I could help set up a clinic at their affiliated orphanage, Casa Alianza, back in Antigua. I had to check with the powers-that-be, but there wasn't a problem. I had been at loose ends in Oratorio, spending most of my time at the refuge anyway.

Whenever I came into Guatemala City from Oratorio, I passed by an elderly lady who lived in a large cardboard box in a doorway. I always gave her a little money. She told me her family lived in a small village outside of the capital and they had brought her to the city because they couldn't afford to take care of her. She had some very bad sores on her legs due to her debilitated health and poor circulation. I always checked her legs and changed the dressings that I got from Peace Corps headquarters. We usually chatted for a while before I wended my way to the refuge or headquarters. I feared she was not the only elderly person brought to the capital city to fend for herself, but I had not seen any other than my box lady. They probably didn't last very long.

I was transferred to Antigua and started working at Casa Alianza, setting up the clinic. I still worked weekends at the refuge in Guatemala City, though, because I missed the children too much.

Father Michael was quietly supportive of birth control in a country of starving people and children thrown away. The Peace Corps supplied its volunteers with as many condoms as they needed or wanted. I always slipped my share to Father Michael, who passed them on to the older boys in the refuge.

There were two older boys whom we had been getting ready to go to school in the capital. They had managed not to get caught up in the paint-sniffing situation and were very bright and personable. Father Michael brought in a tutor from the Antiguan orphanage, and the boys worked very hard at catching up to their grade level. Father Michael gave me some money to take them shopping for school clothes, and we had a lot of fun. It was just like they were my own kids. Of course, they wanted everything they saw, and I wished I could get it all for them. Father Michael and I saw them off to school on their first day. We both fought back tears and agreed that we felt like proud parents.

Before joining the Peace Corps, I had studied martial arts for many years. One day I was browsing in a bookstore in Antigua and noticed a flyer for a karate school. I contacted the instructor and started classes. My karate teacher, Henrik, asked me if I would talk with his wife about prenatal care and childbirth. She was pregnant with their first child and was a little nervous about it. Mirna was an indigenous Indian from a tribe in San Antonio Aguas Calientes, not far from Antigua. They made a delightful couple; he was about six-foot-two and she was somewhere around four-foot-six.

Mirna did not speak English; she spoke her tribal dialect. But she did speak, read, and write Spanish. There was a Peace Corps book, *Where There Is No Doctor*, available in both English and Spanish, so we read the two versions together.

I enjoyed working with Mirna. We went through the pregnancy and childbirth sections of the book in a few weeks and she asked if I would go over the rest of the book with her. She was very intelligent and a pleasure to teach.

Henrik told me a little about his life with Mirna and her tribe, the Q'eq'chi. Mirna's aunt, Rafaela Cordinez, was the chief, so Mirna had a lot of status. When Henrik was dating Mirna, his status with the tribe was very low because he was a *gringo*. After they became formally engaged, their status as a couple increased. They were married in Denmark, Henrik's home country, and then returned to Guatemala to marry in the Q'eq'chi style. Mirna's status then rose to "Wise One," and she became a mother/teacher to the younger members of the tribe.

Several months later, our sessions ended. Mirna said she would continue to study the book and that Henrik would help her if there was anything she didn't understand. I later learned from Henrik that after each of our lessons, Mirna returned to her tribe and conducted classes there, teaching the others what she had learned from me. He said the members of the tribe were questioning some of the old practices, and I had had much influence on the entire Q'eq'chi tribe, with far-reaching consequences.

It touched my heart to know I'd helped children already struggling, and made it safer for babies waiting to be born. For a nurse, it doesn't get any better than that. As my time in the Peace Corps drew to a close, I summarized my lessons. I had learned:

1. How to sleep on the ground and still be able to get up by myself.
2. How to make a good meal out of food I would have thrown away back home.
3. How to take a shower with my shoes on.
4. How to bathe and do other personal things in public.
5. How to feel confident that I am communicating well with other people even when I am not.
6. How to maintain my poise while being body-searched by a teenager with a machine gun.
7. How to give all city thieves a fair share by never getting robbed by the same one twice.
8. Don't get too fond of the pig.

Avenging Vultures

~

Joyce Mueller, RN

Lahore, Pakistan, 1969, the Ford Foundation Guest House:

"Abdul," I called through the screen door.

Karim, not Abdul, hurried out to greet me. "Abdul gone *hakim* shop to get big medicine. He suffer too much in the belly." Karim clutched his own belly. "Poor Abdul," he moaned. He was also moaning for poor Karim, who would be doing all the work himself if Abdul remained too sick to return. And, from Karim's description, he probably was.

"Karim, Karim," I said shaking my head, "don't you remember that any staff members who get sick must come to *memsahib*?"

"*Haguo, memsahib*; we know."

I knew, too, that the Pakistani workers, distrustful of

Western medicos and medicines, preferred to use strong laxatives for their home-remedy cures, no matter what the complaint. These men listened to me only because they needed to keep their jobs. I—a woman, a foreigner, an infidel—supervised their general health and the cleanliness standards essential for keeping our international guests healthy.

I had been volunteered for this job because of my medical background, plus my basic grasp of the culture after four years of living in Pakistan.

"Thanks for helping, Karim. You'll get a bonus," I called back as driver William and I hurried off to find Abdul. We went to the nearest *hakim* shop—the Asian version of a Western pharmacy. It carried everything from ground pearls and dried frog-eyes to strong laxatives and outdated penicillin.

"There he is!" William pointed to a young man wearing a long white shirt and loose pants—the uniform of the guest-house staff.

I could see the telltale brown cascara bottle in his left hand. As he came out the door he suddenly wavered, groaned, and doubled over.

Without thinking, I jumped from the car, pushing aside gawking bystanders, and reached out to keep him from falling. What had I done? A foreign female touching a Muslim man in public!

The gathering crowd began buzzing like a hive of angry bees. Quickly, William stepped in to elbow them away, guiding us to the safety of the car.

"I'm sorry," I said. "Abdul, I meant only to help. You know you are very sick. William will drive you to the hospital right now."

"No, no, *memsahib,* too feared I die in hospital."

"You could die if you don't get treatment. Will you let my doctor examine you? He is a very good doctor." As I spoke, I gently took the bottle of laxatives from him. In too much pain to argue, Abdul let us take him to the hospital.

Outside the doctor's office he balked. "No, *memsahib,* too feared!" But when another spasm struck, he agreed. "But you must also come, *memsahib.*"

The diagnosis of severe liver abscess from amoebiasis meant immediate medical and surgical intervention. Abdul's eyes bulged in terror as he begged me to stay close by.

Poor fella, I thought, he was thinking he was going to die, and he had only me, a female infidel, in whom to put his trust. It was a hard choice for both of us. I certainly didn't want to let him down, but my staying with him presented me with a dangerous problem.

In the culture of his people, my helping him made me "his mama, his papa," responsible for his well-being from then on. If he died as a result of his disease while in my care, the family honor could be satisfied only by taking my life to pay for his—or by the extortion of many, many rupees.

I had made a promise to this fine young man. To leave him now would be unthinkable. His family had been notified of his illness, but they lived several travel days from Lahore in a remote village in the northwest province. With luck, there would be time enough for me, with the help of Karim and William, to nurse Abdul through the first rough days of his illness and still allow me to make my getaway.

On the morning of Abdul's third hospital day, I arrived early at his bedside to find him flat out, stiff, with his eyes closed, looking awfully dead. As I grabbed his wrist to check for a pulse, his eyelids fluttered open. He giggled. He had been feigning death. I was about to scold him when I heard loud whispers and shuffling feet out in the corridor. I glanced at Abdul, who was again playing possum. This confirmed my fears—his family!

They swept toward his bedside like a swarm of starving vultures. Five women, all dressed in black burqas that covered them from head to toe, stopped dead center at the foot of his cot. They stared at me—holding his wrist to check his pulse.

One of the vultures screamed. "*Maut! Maut!* He's dead!" They all began to wail loudly, and the heftiest vulture grabbed my hair to yank me out of the way.

"Abdul," I yelled. "Save me!"

Abdul opened one eye. He smiled wanly, groaned a little, and sighed. What an act! My life was in jeopardy and he was putting on a show.

"Abdul," I hissed.

He opened both eyes, looked directly at my hair-pulling captor, and spoke a few Punjabi words.

She tossed me aside like a broken doll and rushed to his side to smother him with hugs, which empowered the others to do the same.

Good time for a getaway, I thought. However, Big Mama dragged me back to the bed, where Abdul had been propped up like a king, his adoring audience hanging on his every word. The women all turned toward me, smiling. Mama enveloped me in her capacious black-robed arms. As I came up for air, the other ladies began kissing my hands and swarming around me.

"Abdul," I begged, "please call them off."

He said something about "*chai*," so the ladies all trooped out to the corridor to set up stoves they had brought to prepare Abdul's meals.

Soon we were gathered again at Abdul's bedside sipping our chai—sweet Punjabi tea, which had been brewed in the hallway of the United Christian Hospital by smiling, chattering Muslim village ladies.

It was safe now to leave Abdul in the care of his doting family. They were no longer avenging vultures, although they might still consider me "his mama, his papa." I managed to slip away while their attention was momentarily diverted elsewhere.

Six weeks later, Abdul knocked on my door. He had brought me a gift, a pair of gold-thread-embroidered leather slippers. "Made just for you in my village for thank you." Maybe this meant the mama-papa thing had been forgotten. I could only hope.

He *salaamed* his goodbye and walked down the path, but at the gate he turned to me to call, "Thank you—my mama, my papa!" But on his face was a mischievous grin.

Peligro

~

Grace Hatmaker, RN, MSN,
PhD student

Nurse desperately needed for Easter break youth
group trip to Mexico. Bus leaves church parking lot at
4:00 a.m. this Friday.

I REREAD the small bulletin-board ad. Twenty
teens would meet up with the local Mexican teens and
clear brush for a church in mountainous central part
of the country. At the last minute, someone thought it
would be a good idea to bring a nurse along. My years
of emergency department nursing had given me exposure
to multiple medical situations. Some recent camp nursing experience had taught me to improvise with limited
resources. But Mexico? I had my doubts. I had never

ventured into a foreign country. Having recently moved from Pennsylvania to California, I was just beginning to learn about the local California-Mexican culture. What if I ran into something I couldn't handle? What if I got sued? I checked my stockpile of unused vacation days, decided to be brave, and volunteered.

I met with Rob and the three adults organizing the trip. They handed me a battered cardboard first-aid kit— "just in case." The contents included an empty bottle of aspirin dust, a bent pair of tweezers, some small Band-Aids, and three individual antacid packs. Rob gave me a list of the teens and their emergency information but no medical information. Deciding this wouldn't do, I stocked a backpack with the essentials, thanks to a donation box that a local surgeon kept for his annual mission trips: flashlight, gloves, scissors, tape, gauze, tissue, small water bottles, analgesics, antacids, anti-diarrheals, and standing orders for over-the-counters. I called every parent and made medication cards for the teens with allergies, asthma, and other conditions.

After about eight raucous hours south on Interstate 99, we passed San Diego and the bus slowed. The teens grew suddenly silent. We produced documents and inched through the border, passing rifled soldiers. Then we sighted our first real shantytown. Naked children and scrawny dogs played and drank in the same mucky stream in which the women washed clothes. A fire smoldered outside each tin-and-cardboard lean-to. Squatting figures poked at the sparks, swatted flies, and cooked.

The bus bumped along potholed highways, then swayed through rutted lanes and curving dirt roads. Hot dust streamed through our slightly opened windows. In addition, the kids were getting carsick.

By twilight we rolled to a stop. From the shadows, first a few, then a dozen more people approached the bus, shouting. They were happy about our safe arrival and were welcoming us. We soon realized that not one of us spoke Spanish. None of them spoke English. We all had Bibles, but no English-Spanish dictionary. The adults got out of the bus and met with the Mexican adults, trying out their best high-school Spanish. After a late-night feast of beans, tortillas, and sweet, cinnamon-spiced rice water, we sang, prayed, and then collapsed into sleeping bags. Tomorrow we would get to know each other and start working. I fell asleep visualizing carsick kids with cuts and bruises.

A bell clanged through the foggy dawn, signaling breakfast: hot tortillas and rice water. After eating our fill, the adults handed each teen a tool—a pick, an ax, a rake, or a shovel. I was in charge of the first-aid box. After hours of yanking out brush, relocating boulders, and dodging snakes, the teens returned to rinse off under the single cold-water hose trickle and prepared for some fun.

Returning to the main campsite and relieved that nobody was hurt or sick, I discovered that as the nurse, I also had kitchen duty. This turned out to be a bonus job, mostly because I could be sure to be one of few accessing daily hot, soapy water, my hands and arms clean all week. Also, the local ladies had great fun trying out their hot-and-spicy bean variations on me for American teen suitability. Slowly I learned some essential Spanish words: *agua* for water, *muy caliente* for very hot, *dolor* for pain/hurt/sick, and *el baño* for the bathroom.

The teens split up into groups, with half American and half Mexican teens on each side. I settled under a tree on a soft spot of dirt, my first-aid kit unused. Anyone who was "sent to the nurse" mostly needed a time-out in the shade or access to the water dribbling from the extension hose, and then ran back to play. A little boy, maybe five or so, walked up to me from a nearby farm. His mother was hanging clothes on a line and singing. His father was strapped behind a mule, pushing a huge stick in front of him to break up the rocky soil.

The boy poked me on the arm and said, "*Peligro.*"

I smiled back, "Yes." I had no clue what he had just said.

"*No*," he said, wrinkling up his little forehead, "*peligro!*"

He looked worried. I scanned all the teens playing ball and said, "Yes, *peligro.*" I sensed he was worried about something, maybe about the teens playing ball? He ran back to his mother, who brushed him away.

He darted back. "*Peligro!*" he insisted.

I patted the soft dirt next to me, raising a small cloud of dust. "Here, sit down and watch. The kids are having fun!"

His black-brown eyes widened as he stepped back, biting his lip and obviously thinking intently. Then he suddenly ran toward me, grabbed me just below the hem of my shorts, and pinched me hard. He ran away from me. "*Peligro!*" he shouted, stomping his foot.

I jumped up. "What did you do that for?" I waved my finger at him. "You hurt me!"

Tears filled his eyes. He pointed with all his might at the soft pad of dirt I had been sitting on. A stream of minuscule red ants poured out of the top of the hill. "*Peligro!*" he insisted. Then I remembered some of the words the kitchen ladies had taught me.

"*Dolor?*" I asked, using the word for "pain."

"*Sí!*"

"*Caliente?*" I asked, for "hot."

Hmmm, he had to think about that. "*Sí!*"

"*Peligro?*" Danger?

He smiled, realizing I had finally understood. Very shortly, I would have been the first to dig through my first-aid box to find some treatment for fire-ant bites. I took the little doe-eyed boy to the kitchen ladies, where he excitedly told them the story of rescuing this American lady nurse from the fire ants. They clucked and patted about him, and gave us both a congratulatory cup of *horchata*, which I later learned was that delicious, sweet cinnamon/vanilla rice water. We walked back hand-in-hand, and Paulo tried very hard to teach me some more Spanish.

After this trip to Mexico, I have ventured out to many other experiences. As a nurse, I would encourage other nurses to consider stepping slightly outside their comfort zones. We can draw from our natural flexibility and holistic approach to healthcare, remember the basics, and provide competent and ethical interventions with good judgment as needed. We can assess, teach, role-model health habits, and treat injuries and illnesses.

Providing nursing care in other cultures, though, can be full of surprising experiences, and I personally grew every time I experienced another way of life and thinking. Every time I return from a trip, I realize that I have received so much more than I gave.

I was humbled watching the daily routine of Paulo's family in the mountains of Mexico. I was overwhelmed by the love and attentiveness of the local kitchen staff. They cooked American-style beans (not too spicy) and *horchata,* extra sweet.

I realized, even without a dictionary, that so much communication is universal. Expressions, gestures, laughter, singing, and playing are a common language. The heart of nursing is sincere caring and sharing our personal gifts and skills. And I believe people around the world sense this.

Don't Be a Wimp

~

Janet M. Vogt, RNFA, BSN, CNOR

T HE PEDIATRIC SURGEON that I work with, Doug, and I went on an investigative trip for International Volunteers (IVU) in Urology to Ulaanbaatar, Mongolia, to see what their pediatric urology needs were. We were hosted by the pediatric surgeon at the Women's and Children's Hospital. She explained what types of urology problems and conditions the local doctors needed help with and the numbers of children who would be needing our help if IVU sent a full team to this location.

Our van ride into the city from the Two Gates airport took us past cattle and sheep grazing freely on the hillsides. We knew we were entering Ulaanbaatar when our vehicle passed through a large, very ornate archway overlooking the city below. At first there were scattered houses, eventually leading to very populated city streets. Our home for the stay would be a previous Czech embassy converted into a bed-and-breakfast for visitors to the country.

While we were there we planned on doing a few surgical cases to check out what the hospital/surgery resources were and how patients were managed. It was mid-September, and it had already snowed the first night of our visit. Upon entering the operating room, I quickly realized the wooden window frames were not sealed well, and cold air was flowing into the room. I had just my scrubs on, no extra T-shirt underneath, so it didn't take long for me to get chilled. All of the local people seemed oblivious to my situation. As we scrubbed for surgery, the scrub nurse took a cloth gown out of a sterile silver canister and placed it on me. As I slipped my arms into the sleeves, I realized it was still damp. The combination of chilly room and damp gown was an awakening experience. I was hoping the case would not last too long. Doug, however, received a disposable paper surgical gown that he ripped off at the end of the surgery.

Back at our rooms later that evening, we discussed the events of the day. I mentioned the gown incident and Doug told me to stop being such a wimp. I retaliated by telling him that some little Mongolian woman was probably sewing his paper gown back together to use tomorrow.

We had noticed how much the people conserved and recycled in this very modest country. In the operating room, that meant that they wasted nothing. Any suture that wasn't used was gathered to be resterilized, no matter how short it was. Needles of all types were collected. Even the used surgical sponges were saved to be laundered and re-sterilized. These practices made me realize just how wasteful we are in Western society. I know we are lucky that we don't need to practice in these extreme ways, but it still makes me aware that we could do more, waste less, and think about whether we really need as much as we think we do.

Their surgical equipment and instruments were not the most up-to-date. They obviously used everything until it could not possibly be fixed or rigged up to work in some fashion. We noticed some nicer equipment (X-ray machines and a portable ultrasound machine) just pushed back in a storage area. When we asked our host about the pieces, we were told they were donated by companies in the United States. However, the machines no longer worked because no one knew how to fix them, and parts were impossible to obtain. So, once something broke, that was the end of its usefulness.

Our hosts, very creative people that they are, took excellent care of their patients in spite of the lack of resources. The padding on the operating room tables and stirrups was almost nonexistent—however, the medical personnel managed to make sure patients had blankets or some sort of padding to prevent positioning problems. They didn't have safety straps, but reused Ace wraps to keep the children secured while asleep. The operating room lights were not hung from the ceiling, but were on stands that had to be moved in close to the OR table. Even placed nearby, their intensity was not much more than that of a good flashlight. However, there were very large windows to allow all the natural light in—so much for working after dark! X-ray view boxes were few and far between. Most of the time the films were taped onto the windows for viewing.

Back in the operating room the second day, my revenge was sweet. As we dressed for the surgery of the day, the scrub nurse gowned Doug with a damp cloth gown. As the chill started to overcome him, his eyes just got bigger and bigger. I leaned over and quietly reminded him, "Don't be a wimp."

Our trip was very informative, both professionally and personally. We learned not only about the country's health needs, but also a lot about the Mongolian people and their culture. The physical characteristics of the Mongolian people remind me of the U.S.'s Native American population. Our hosts showed us around the capital city of Ulaanbaatar and then out to the countryside. My favorite part of our country tour was a visit to a replica of the Genghis Khan base camp and hunting skills arena. These people are very proud of their heritage. The visit would not have been complete without a trip to the cashmere factory. Doug and I both knew our families would be impressed with our choice of gifts for them.

I have returned to Mongolia three times since that initial investigative trip. I continue to fall deeper in love with the people each time. Every trip I see more, learn more, and appreciate my own life and family much more. During my last trip, a close family member passed away.

My host co-workers comforted me as if they had known me all my life. They worked diligently, making phone calls and arrangements so I would be able to leave two days before the rest of my group. They made it possible for me to arrive home in time for the services, a gesture I will never forget.

Our hosts, in any of the countries I have visited on medical mission trips, are always very appreciative of our skills and care for their patients. But the truth is, I know I receive much more than I could possibly do for them in the short time we are with them.

Always Pack White Underwear

~

Sarah Liberman, RN, MSN

As you get ready to go abroad, there are always numerous people ready with advice to assist you. One friend mentioned plastic baggies as an indispensible travel item; another recommended good walking shoes that have been broken in. I heeded this advice and stuffed my giant cherry-red suitcase full of power bars, a fancy dress (just in case), and lots of extra pairs of socks.

I was working on my bachelor's of science in nursing in Saskatchewan and was going to finish my degree by completing my two final practicums in Helsinki, Finland. I had never imagined I would end up in Scandinavia. I did suffer from delusions of grandeur when it came to travel, but they were mostly situated in India or Africa—a place where everything would be so different. Little did I know that the place that seemed to be the most like home would teach me so much.

I applied for the Finland placement because it was three months in duration and fairly independent. I would need to rent an apartment, and essentially learn how to live in another context. While I would have a faculty contact, and be placed with nurse mentors, rather than be in a group of people all the time I would take the bus to work, buy my own groceries, and wash my own laundry.

I arrived in Finland very excited, and promptly found how huge my luggage seemed for how small European cars were. My Finnish education continued as I went to get groceries. In Finland, as with most of Europe, you weigh and label your vegetables before you bring them to the register. I learned this only *after* being yelled at in Finnish and then in Swedish, which was finally translated to me in English by another customer. I learned my lesson and started shopping with my language book so I could identify the right word for a *kurkku* (cucumber) and ensure it was weighed and labeled. I was late for my first day at the hospital, not knowing that you have to flag your bus down just like you would a taxi. Sleepy-eyed and jet-lagged, I had to miss a couple buses before watching a Finnish person clued me in to this practice.

When I arrived at the hospital, I met the nurses and was given a tour of the intensive-care burns unit, which is where I would spend the next six weeks. The unit was smaller than the ones I was used to but was comparable to a general ICU at home. The nurses were very friendly, and the cafeteria had great lunches. I exhaled, relieved that I could get my meals here and decrease my presence at the local grocery store. (I was still traumatized by my recent multilingual instruction/scolding.) Since this was an ICU, scrubs were supplied and laundered by the hospital. I am not sure it showed but I blanched a little when they showed me my options: thin, white scrubs. I know white is traditional for nurses, but at home no one ever wore white scrubs. They get so dirty, and there are so many other colors to choose from.

It wasn't that wearing white bothered me, however old-school I perceived it to be. It was that while I was heeding the advice of my better-traveled friends, no one mentioned that I would need white underwear. At home that night I looked through my suitcase and found a fatal flaw in my affection for bright, crazy undergarments, including my favorite pair, bright-green polka-dotted underwear with hot-pink lace trim. Of course, I could go to the store to buy some white underwear. However, Finland is an expensive country, and I had maxed out my student line of credit just to get there and pay my rent.

The next day, it took about five minutes before the first colleague of mine commented on my underwear. I was mortified, and could imagine failing my practicum because of unprofessional attire. I did the best I could, trying to ensure that I wore the most subtle colors on shift, and that laundry happened on a regular basis. Most of the people I worked with laughed and thought of it as a funny quirk of mine. Perhaps it even helped me make friends, something that was somewhat difficult. Finland is a bilingual country, much like Canada, with the two languages being Finnish and Swedish. This meant talking with me involved a third language, and people's discomfort with that language could often make them shy away from conversation.

Some clients spoke excellent English, learned from watching undubbed American television programs. Others would try to speak Spanish to me, assuming from my dark hair and eyes that I must be from Spain, a common vacation spot.

One client I cared for during most of my clinical rotation barely spoke any English. He had very bad burns from jumping out of a second-floor window when his house caught fire. The extensive burns required hours of wound care and close observation. I spent many hours by Toumas's bedside, monitoring vital signs and ensuring that he was comfortable and his pain was under control.

It was one dressing change with Toumas that changed how I felt about being a nurse. Throughout school I had focused mainly on learning and mastering the various nursing skills. Often, as students, we had contributed to the care of other nurse's clients if it enabled us to try a task for the first time. The dressing changes were very painful for the client as he healed, and despite pain medication, some discomfort seemed unavoidable. During one particularly painful and detailed dressing change, I decided to stay by the head of the bed and hold his hand. The nurses were able to communicate quicker if they didn't need to speak English, and I felt that someone needed to be with the client as he was hoisted up on his side, being poked and prodded by a team of professionals.

Toumas was aware that I was a foreign nursing student, and in broken English he said it was okay if I left him and went to the other side to be with the nurses. His comments made me see that he understood the severity of the burns and felt that I should be able to see them. I had had burns myself from an accident years before, and knew not only the physical pain but also the emotional pain that was a part of the body disfigurement scar tissue can cause. I politely let him know that it was okay, and if he would agree, I would rather stay there with him.

It was a few minutes before I realized he was crying. Later, he told one of the nurses that it meant so much to him that had I stayed to comfort him. What I learned at that moment was that it didn't matter that I had to flag down buses, weigh my vegetables, or wear white underwear; some things were the same no matter what culture you are in. People need to be treated as people, and nurses have an amazing opportunity to ensure that this happens. In the middle of ICU wards, where multiple machines, lines, and leads are hooked up to unstable patients, it can be tough to think about the pieces of us that can't be measured through vital signs.

When my time in Finland ended, as I packed my bag to go home, I reflected on the tears that had rolled down Toumas's face. I now had my own piece of advice to give colleagues when they prepared for their own excursions into international nursing: pack white underwear, and always remember that caring is transcultural.

PART FOUR

Looking Back

The State of Emergency

~

Paula Nangle, RN, BA, MFA

CHRISTIAAN BARNARD performed the world's first heart transplant at Groote Schuur Hospital in Cape Town, South Africa. My mother believed she dazzled people with this fact. When I trained there, it was a rambling building without central heat—damp in winter, the worst in July, when patients would shiver during bed baths. I would huddle up inside my cape on tea breaks. Inside and out, perhaps since it had a lit turret, the building reminded me of a turn-of-the-century state hospital in northern Michigan, and I felt for it a similar awe.

Because of apartheid, Groote Schuur used to be segregated by race. When I dream of the hospital now, it is always a dream of mazes—familiar halls to Non-White and White wings, and all the underground tunnels. Most often I see the long tunnel up Table Mountain to the nurses' home, and its blood-red tile. There was a ceiling beaded with water that never dripped, and echoey footsteps of soled shoes, going up and going down—thundering groups of nurses on their way to Report at 0:650 a.m. Or my own steps, which in my dream are really the erratic beating of my heart. I recall porters—merry white men in protected jobs—running the box gurneys up the tunnel to the morgue. The gurneys, called trolleys, would rattle and echo, and the porters would laugh above the din with a nervous hilarity.

It was 1982. I had flunked out of Michigan State in my junior year. My father and mother, missionaries in Zimbabwe, flew me back to Africa on a diminished travel fund. Their supporting churches prayed. I had spent much of my last year in East Lansing taking speed provided by various boyfriends. The last one had told me, blowing smoke rings, to *have a good life*. I felt humiliated and contrite. At the same time, I believed I could "do something" to change South Africa—an odd notion, considering how I'd squandered my time in college. I knew nothing about nurses' training and originally didn't care. Family friends helped organize a work permit. Every six months I presented myself at Immigration down on the Waterfront, and an Afrikaans-speaking clerk would stamp my passport. I adapted.

My mother said the structure was good for me. It was true, it seemed. I liked adding new stripes to my epaulettes each time I finished a three-month block. I had five blocks—times of lectures and tests—to finish before I got my pin. I loved these tangible ways of proving my knowledge, and how I could wear the stripes, flaunt them, and practice new responsibilities with them. Between blocks I did my rotations, 12-hour shifts on days or nights, in assigned wards. The student nurses worked as aides, although I passed medications after the first four months. I proudly pushed the cart around a Florence Nightingale wing. The hard work suited me. I thrived on basic ways of helping afflicted patients. I learned to make prioritizing lists—feeding tubes, the dressing trolley, and the sterile technique to prevent staphylococcus. I could relieve someone's pain in a matter of minutes with morphine and Panado. Aside from doing dressings, or treating Isolation patients, we never used gloves, even while washing bedpans. My entire world that first year was made up of learned tasks. I realized I could provide comfort, and this came to me as a surprise.

Starting in the mid-1980s, South Africa was faced with increased popular resistance to apartheid and violent township protests, which led the government to declare a State of Emergency. In 1985, President P.W. Botha announced that violence in the country showed that "ordinary law and order was inadequate." The State of Emergency gave more powers to the police and military and prevented the media from covering unrest.

I worked B11 Theater during the *State of Emergency*. On night shift, the nurses—most of B11's permanent night staff were African and mixed-race—could be called out to any theater in the hospital. While waiting for the phone to ring, I would doze with them under bunny blankets, or we would smoke and talk. They taught me names for the surgeons who threw instruments. One was called *nat broek*, "wet diaper."

To wake up for the next surgery, we would hand each other warm cloths, *yamalappies*, and freshen our faces. It was a month of bizarre sights. I counted swabs. I was expected to hold buckets for discarded pieces of bowel and teeming intestinal worms. Once I caught a dismembered foot. I followed orders and could run fast to the central supply dispensary for specially autoclaved packs. It felt like a kind of break for me, standing there not having to think, while the scrub sister and surgeon made life-and-death decisions.

One night, the Accident Unit sent us a number of stabbings. Unrest out in Guguletu, we were told. Masked surgeons moved from theater to theater. Between our assigned surgeries, Sister Cloete and I and the other student, Miriam, paced around the break room and smoked. The other nurses rushed in between their assignments, flushing the toilet, smoking, and eating. One of the stab victims lay on a trolley out in the hall and would ask us for a *stompie* every time we walked by. Sister Cloete rolled out on her chair and held her cigarette for him.

"He needs a dressing change," she told me.

I applied Betadine and some four-by-fours (gauze bandages) to the hole in his chest, caused, he told me, by a Phillips-head screwdriver. I taped it. He kept asking me for water. "I'm sorry," I told him, he was NPM—nil per mouth. He needed to rest and wait for his operation, I said.

He knew English. When I asked, he told me he lived in Khayalitsha. He lay there on the trolley outside the break room and looked around. He was long and thin; his feet hung over the end of the trolley, and he kept flexing and relaxing his toes. He shivered at times. I covered him with a warm blanket from the warmer. Sister Cloete assigned some of the staff to sit near him whenever they were free because she thought he might take something from their handbags. Or he might stand up and walk away.

"And he will surely die in that case," she said. "That puncture wound is deep."

Hours later, after we returned from the treating the hematoma, the man was still there. We all took turns watching him, rolling back and forth in and out of the break room. He began muttering the Xhosa word *sela*, which might have meant either "drink" or "thief." It reminded me of a word I liked and never understood in Psalms—*selah*. But certainly he meant "drink." I became thirsty watching him. I held my cigarette to his dry lips. Near dawn, I could hear the slamming of pans and instruments onto trolleys. An unconscious patient rolled past us to Recovery.

"You're next now," I told the man.

Sister Cloete must have taken him into the holding room, because Miriam and I were summoned to C11 Theater to wrap a body. The dead man seemed much younger than the screwdriver victim, around my age, maybe even a boy in his teens, although he had no Identity Document—the controversial pass he was required by Pass Laws to carry.

A sister asked me to label the body bag "xxxx" with the time of death, 0600. No one had time to tell us the whole story. The young man had been stabbed, pronounced brain-dead, and kept alive on the ventilator. His heart had been used for a transplant in the adjoining theater. I could hear the other ventilator in the next room.

There was a large bandage across the deceased man's chest, thickly taped with Elastoplast (a bandage that stretches). His eyes had been removed and sutured. Miriam and I knew how to wrap bodies. This task was always left for students, and sometimes we complained about it. When we finished taping him up, we left him on the table. The C11 sister invited us to watch the transplant. We stood in the doorway to the next room, crowded with masked professionals of unknown rank, a group of surgeons and anesthesiologists near the sterile green tents. I understood that the bewildering mass of tubes was the heart-lung machine. I turned back to watch a porter lift the man's body into a box trolley. I wondered where the man would go after the morgue.

I thought of my father. He would have been asking about the patient's religion, likely trying to pray over him. It would have been a good question, I had to admit. And who would be looking for this man? How would they find him? I felt tired on my feet and asked the sister if I could return to B11.

When I think now of this particular transplant, I wonder about forms, consents, documentation—red tape. It seems that filling out forms is all I do on certain workdays. "There's a form for everything," my co-workers and I will say to one another, usually rolling our eyes. For organ donation, I attend a mandatory in-service every year. There is a person to call to talk to the family. I am an organ donor, and to obtain a sticker for my driver's license I had to fill out an online application. I speculate now about the laws in South Africa back then. I have never thought to find out what the law was, or whether there might have been special provisions for unusual circumstances. Or possibly a consent had been taken care of—it might have been only a rumor that the man was found without a Pass, and there had been some other reason for writing "xxxx" on the bag—confidentiality, perhaps. My assumptions, even then, and in that place at that time, vaguely disgust me.

Back in B11, the other man's surgery was already over. Aides and students were wiping up blood and dusting the diathermy machine (a medical instrument for local heating of bodily tissues for medical purposes). The man with the screwdriver in his chest had not survived. He'd died almost immediately on the table, and, to my relief, someone had already wrapped him. Sister Cloete stood in the break room. She was ripping off her scrubs and getting into her uniform and raincoat for the train out to Mitchell's Plain.

"Cardiac tamponade," she said to me (a clinical syndrome caused by the accumulation of fluid in the pericardial space—the sac around the heart).

"But he seemed fine," I said. "I had no idea."

Sister Cloete crouched in front of the mirror to bobby-pin her cap. "Lying around on a trolley all night?" She gestured with her hands. "No. No, I won't say anything. Surely you don't believe we had such a shortage of surgeons in the house."

"I'm glad we let him smoke those two cigarettes," I said as I handed Sister Cloete her umbrella.

"You know, then," she said. "His last comfort, I suppose."

Fifteen years later, my husband and I visited Cape Town. We toured the Robben Island Museum. We drove up to the old Groote Schuur, parking in a ramp outside the new hospital. A man offered to watch our car for a fee. It was raining in a typical way. No one appeared to be around except a woman mopping floors in the old Accident Unit. We walked through the main door. It had never been much of an entranceway. We climbed the stairs to C2 Orthopedic—offices now. No one else was around. On B floor, we saw that B11 had become a museum for heart transplants. We read the sign. I thought this mildly odd, since it seemed to me that heart transplants were always done on C11, and I mentioned this to my husband. On the day we visited, it happened to be a public holiday we didn't know about, and the double doors to B11 were locked with a chain. I tried to peer through the crack into the dark space. I could not say what it was that I wanted— to open the door, I suppose, on what I'd only peripherally seen and never quite appreciated one time inside the walls of this old building. Still now, with its smell of rot and Dettol, I felt a kind of shame in the longing.

Journey to the
Mekong Delta

~

Cheri Clark, RN

IT WAS the summer of 1974, just weeks after we had set up the Friends of Children of Vietnam (FCVN) Adoption Center in Saigon. Vietnam was in the grips of one of the deadliest wars in modern history. As a recently graduated registered nurse, I had come to volunteer my help.

As inevitably happens in war, it was the children who suffered the most. The purpose of FCVN was to care for and offer hope to the most vulnerable of those children, the orphans—often abandoned within hours of birth by young mothers, driven to desperation by a combination of crushing poverty and social stigma.

Many of these abandoned children were the products

of brief unions between young, unwed Vietnamese women and young American soldiers. These were the children who were most at risk due to the enormous social stigma of such unions. Often, they were children so unwanted that they had no names.

Just weeks after setting up the adoption center in Saigon, I made my first trip into the famous Mekong Delta. It was a journey that I will never forget, taking me through scenes that remain vividly etched in my memory to this day—for they were scenes that were to repeat themselves over and over, and become a familiar motif in my life.

We rented a van and driver for our journey. It was an old beat-up Ford with no air conditioning that looked as if it wouldn't even make it across the city. We loaded up the diapers, medicine, food, and some clothing, and embarked on the risky journey to the Delta.

As we left the relative security of Saigon behind, the mounting evidence of military activity was a stark reminder of the war being fought in the areas we were visiting. Only a few miles outside the city we came face-to-face with the Vietnamese Army.

Tanks stood menacingly by small roadside encampments, heavy machine-gun barrels jutted out from sandbag encampments, and the entire area was surrounded with rolls of barbed wire. Soldiers seemed to be everywhere, on tanks and in guard posts. Some were still sleeping in hammocks slung in nearby trees, and even underneath military trucks.

As we progressed southward toward the Delta, the military presence increased dramatically. Heavily armed soldiers guarded each turn in the road. Jeeps and military trucks, all painted in drab green camouflage, were parked alongside the road, and soldiers watched our slow progress.

When we came upon a long army convoy, we were forced to creep at a snail's pace behind it. These convoys were prime targets for Viet Cong rockets. In spite of the military all around us and the undercurrent of imminent danger, I felt a deep sense of purpose and a certain exhilaration to be making such a journey.

The countryside was a vast vista of fields filled with greenery. The landscape was dotted with tombs that at first glance seemed to have been placed haphazardly in almost every field. Thuy, a Vietnamese social worker, explained that the farmers and their families buried their dead in their own fields whenever possible. It was a strange sight for my Western eyes, and the large number of new graves was a grim reminder of the war zone through which we were driving.

Hours later we reached the Mekong River and stopped behind a long line of vehicles waiting to board a ferry. The embarkation area was packed solid with vehicles and foot passengers, all jostling for space on the old wooden ferry. Every square inch of the ferry was packed like sardines in a can with hot, sweating, noisy humanity.

After a hectic disembarkation at the other end, we made it back onto the asphalt road to continue our drive to the first orphanage. By now, we had lapsed into a listless silence; we just wanted to reach our destination and start our planned visits.

We made our first stop at Diem Phuc, an orphanage just outside Vinh Long, which we hoped would become the next addition to FCVN's Foster Orphanage Project. After greetings and the customary unsweetened, lukewarm tea, we entered the orphanage for a quick tour.

The rooms where the older children lived were crowded. The nursery was in a tiny room upstairs. Inside, we saw several girls in charge of about 20 babies. The air smelled of dirt and disease. I walked past cribs filled with sick babies lying in rough, dirty diapers. Their bodies were red and sore, and they were so wasted away that their bones were visible through their skin.

Another small room held perhaps 50 children of toddler age. The children lay in cribs with wooden slat bases; there were no mattresses to cushion their frail bodies. The toddlers wore no diapers and their urine and feces dropped through the slats to the filthy floor, which obviously had not been cleaned for at least hours, maybe days.

The room was full of flies that flew from piles of waste to the babies' faces, no doubt spreading infection throughout the room. Seeing the conditions in the orphanage, it was no surprise to me that many of these places had a mortality rate of 80 percent.

I was drawn to two African-American children lying in a corner crib. I reached into the crib and examined them before picking one of them up. She was too weak to hold her head up, and she rested quietly against my shoulder. Next to her, the other black child was burning with fever, her eyes glazed and tormented.

"What are their names?" I asked. The sister gestured toward the sick baby in the crib and said her name was Minh Trang; the other child, she said, shrugging toward the baby in my arms, had no name.

I learned that both of the girls had been abandoned just after their births. I decided that when we passed on our way back to Saigon, I would ask the director to allow them to go back with us.

Next, we visited the Good Shepherd Orphanage in Vinh Long. The grounds were immaculate, the sisters cheerful, and the children clean, well stimulated, and healthy. Sister Ursula, a nun from Malaysia who seemed to have a permanent smile on her face, escorted us through a very clean, well-run nursery.

Although we were in a hurry to leave before nightfall, when the fighting would recommence, the sisters encouraged us to take the time to stop at yet another orphanage, St. Paul's, also in Vinh Long. They told us that the orphanage was poor, but despite the lack of funding the staff took excellent care of the children.

We took the nuns' advice and soon found St. Paul's, where we arrived unexpectedly. St. Paul's director, Sister Marie Christine, was eager to tell us about her orphanage. After tea, we were ushered into a large, baby-filled nursery. An elderly nun led us past each crib and gave us a running commentary about each baby; it was obvious she knew each child personally.

The sisters confided that they had to water down the children's daily formula so there would be enough to go around. At night, they had only rice water to feed the babies. Thuy and I agreed that we should start helping these sisters, who were doing so much with so little. We walked to our van and gave freely of our dwindling supplies. Before we left, keen to cross in the next ferry before it stopped running at dusk, the nuns asked us to take some of their babies to Saigon, and we agreed to call in on our return trip.

It was dark when we arrived at the Providence Orphanage in Can Tho, the southernmost point of my first trip to the Mekong Delta. Sister Eugenia, the director, greeted us with a bright smile and a warm welcome.

The children were all asleep and the building was quiet. The nuns showed us to the guest quarters at the top of the spindly staircase. The guest room was simple but clean. The nuns had kindly carried in buckets of water, and I thankfully shed my dirty clothes and washed down. Just being clean and wearing fresh clothes seemed a luxury after spending the day cooped up in the hot, dusty van.

We ate an evening meal with all the sisters. We all chatted for a while, and the sisters told us of other orphanages, deeper in the Delta, that were even more desperate for help. These orphanages were rarely visited by any outside agencies; they were overloaded with infants and their resources were stretched to the breaking point.

When I went up to bed and lay in darkness, the war seemed very close. I could hear gunfire and the noise of rockets being fired in the nearby jungle, exploding with loud crashes. Tired after a long journey, I fell asleep to the sounds of war.

The next day I woke up early. The older children were already up and about, laughing as they prepared to go to school. I saw them running around the yard and playing on the swings and slides. It was a far cry from some of the orphanages I'd seen in Saigon.

The baby room was small but clean. The babies slept in little hammocks suspended over their cribs, to keep them cooler. Each crib was decorated with colorful mobiles. Despite the good care, many of the babies were very sick. The sisters explained that sometimes as many as 20 babies would arrive in a single week. Often they had been abandoned in the maternity hospital, where they lay unattended for several days before arriving at the orphanage, sick and dehydrated.

Outside the nursery, we saw bookshelves filled with photograph albums of children who had left the orphanage and been adopted. The pictures attested to the nuns' belief in adoption. They knew that the adoptees were likely to become bright and healthy in their new lives, unlike many of the sick and dying that remained behind.

Before we left, the sisters asked us to take four infants with us to Saigon. Three of them were tiny baby boys and the other was a little girl named Kim Hoa, with thick black hair and lovely eyes. She had a cleft lip and palate, which we knew could easily be repaired by doctors in America.

After giving out the last of our supplies, we laid several blankets on the floor at the back of the van. Thuy and I would sit on the floor and care for the babies during the long drive back to Saigon. We said a hurried farewell to the sisters and promised to return soon.

Once we were on the road, Thuy and I named the boys. All four infants were in poor physical shape; all were less than a week old and only one weighed more than five pounds. The journey was slow and the hot sun was beginning to dehydrate the sickest of our charges. Waiting for the ferry, we were forced to sit in the heat, watching the life slowly ebbing from our four babies. We managed to get the attention of somebody in authority and finally—after waiting a couple of hours for an important military convoy to be ferried across—we were given priority and took the next boat over the river.

As promised the day before, we stopped at St. Paul's. The sisters had four babies for us to take. We now had eight tiny babies to care for on the road to Saigon, and we still had one more stop to make. The nuns had tears in their eyes as they bade farewell to the little ones they were entrusting to our care.

We hurried on to Diem Phuc, the first orphanage we had visited the day before. The director had returned from Saigon and greeted us warmly. We asked her if we could take the half-American children back to Saigon with us. The director looked at the other babies in the van and had a brief discussion with some of the other nuns.

A few minutes later the director and some other nuns arrived, carrying the two half-American girls we had seen the previous day. The director motioned for one of the tired sisters to give Minh Trang to Thuy. She explained that the child had a fever again. Another nun handed me the other baby, and we carefully set them side-by-side on the blankets we had laid on the floor. Thuy told the sisters that I wanted to name the little girl after my own adopted child. The nuns nodded enthusiastically at my suggestion, and so Thu Loan was named.

We thanked the director and promised to do our best for the children. By now the heat of the day was building and the temperature inside the van was climbing even higher. We started our journey homeward.

The last leg of the long journey was dreadful as we sat on the floor, fed the babies, and cared for the sick ones among them. By then the babies were uncomfortable and in need of proper medical attention. Driving along a bumpy road in the hot van was extracting a high price from them.

As we finally pulled up the driveway of the adoption center in Saigon, my colleagues and the nursery staff rushed out to greet us, happy to see us safe and well after our trip into the Delta. When they looked into the van and saw Thuy and me surrounded by so many tiny babies, they were taken aback. We had brought ten children, eight of them infants less than a month old, many of them sick and in need of urgent care. The children were whisked off to the nursery.

And now, each of them had a name.

One Born on a Rainy Day

~

Michele J. Upvall, PhD, RN, FNP

IT'S A RAINY DAY in Africa and I'm awakened by the sound of an infant. I can hear the sound of the pounding rain on the tin roof and see the pellets of water smacking against the coverless window on another hopeful African pre-dawn. Feeling groggy and confused, I look from my bed to the left of the room where a newborn, as angry as the rain on the windows, is crying for her mother. This is my baby and she's waiting for me to welcome her.

In 1989, the year she was born, Swaziland was a country with all the deadly issues facing other underdeveloped parts of the world. Respiratory infections, diarrheal diseases, malaria, and more were prevalent in a country with few resources to manage them and were especially devastating for the children. Then the pandemic of HIV/AIDS arrived, which Swaziland had only begun to battle when we returned in 1992. Two full years in Swaziland, although interrupted by a two-year period, only intensified my desire to work as a nurse with a global perspective.

The Kingdom of Swaziland lies in southern Africa, bordered on three sides by the Republic of South Africa with Mozambique to the northeast. Atypical of many African countries ruled by foreign powers from 1800 through the 1900s, Swaziland retained its monarchy to govern the mostly homogeneous ethnic group, the Swazis, when Britain decolonized it in 1968.

This lush, little-known kingdom, with only 6,700 square miles, also welcomed this new baby whom the midwives named Lomvula, or "One born on a rainy day." A sign of good luck, they told me. We were not off to the most auspicious start, however. The nurses were eager for me to wake up after general anesthesia from a cesarean section to feed her. From baby Lomvula's cry, it was known to all that the spoonfuls of sugar water they patiently provided would not appease her.

It was not my intention to have a baby in a place so far from my home in Pennsylvania. In fact, I wasn't sure having a baby would ever be in my future. I simply hadn't thought about it much, since my first priority was to complete my doctoral dissertation.

My love for nursing began when I was young, and reading the story of "A Ship Called HOPE" encouraged me to think of nursing as a career that could serve the world. Professors in nursing and anthropology encouraged me in my dreams, allowing me to seek independent study credits in Nigeria on Christmas break while working on my Bachelor of Science in Nursing. During that trip in 1985 I experienced my first coup, a military overthrow of President Shehu Shagari. A few years later, Swaziland provided a coup of a different sort.

I will never know how Swaziland became the subject of my dissertation. Did I choose it, or did it choose me? Traditional healing methods had always intrigued me; so when I read about a traditional healer in Swaziland working with nurses to provide primary healthcare teaching to the country's large numbers of healers, who in turn would teach their patients, I was even more curious. How could nurses and traditional healers from such very different belief systems work together, and what implications could this have on the health of the country? Off I went to find out, getting married along the way in the hills of Siteki, in the smallest topographical region of Swaziland.

My days were occupied with ethnographic research and overcoming the many stumbling blocks along the way that you can never truly prepare for when conducting research in another country. The traditional healer helped me navigate Swaziland's political system by introducing me to the minister of health, who provided the necessary documents for me to show my research participants. The informed-consent letter from my home university was useless in my new home. Clearly, the required telephone numbers for the Institutional Review Board from the university would not work in a country where telephones could be difficult to find, even for those who could pay the charges.

Documents in hand, off I went, working with a nurse in a private physician's office to learn the language of nursing in Swaziland. After a few months, it was time to explore with the public health nurses. As I traveled with them over dusty roads, in Jeeps filled with medicines and equipment to immunize and weigh the children, I began to understand their culture.

Conversation was polite and they answered my endless questions with patience, teaching me the art of nursing in a land of few resources and far too many obstacles. It was not, however, until they discovered that I was going to have a baby of my own that they truly recognized me as more than an outsider, a researcher with little in common with them as nurses and as women. Before my pregnancy, I was a stranger—even worse, a youngster, in their eyes, who was far away from home and family, a situation unimaginable within their culture.

Having a baby during the research process made me realize the human element that can profoundly impact research in a way that I'd never considered. Connecting with others at a deeply personal level provided richness to the dialogue between me and those taking part in my study, both nurses and traditional healers. Even though I was without the gray hair that would command more immediate respect within a culture that values its elderly, I still had a common bond with the women who informed the study. Their eyes lit up when I told them of my pregnancy, and they were eager to share stories of their own childbirth and Swazi customs surrounding pregnancy and birth. Their words came from their hearts, as I was now "more like them."

Yet the differences between us as women were significant. Their value as women was enhanced through childbearing, and even the king of Swaziland could not be considered married until pregnancy had occurred. Customs that I recall to ensure a healthy pregnancy were mostly concerned with preventing supernatural causes of illness. Avoiding lightning at all costs was considered extremely important. Also, staying indoors late in the day, near sunset, prevented harm to the baby from sorcerers. Various herbs were given to pregnant women by traditional birth attendants (TBAs) to prevent breech delivery, as well as to accelerate labor. Nurses did not admit to taking these herbs during their own pregnancies, but did share stories of caring for women who died during labor from using these natural oxytocics (substances that stimulate the uterus to contract).

Expectations during childbirth differed as well. Women in labor were to remain stoic and quiet, despite the pain. This was not a goal that I believed I could easily accomplish! Many of the Swazi women preferred to deliver their babies at home in the presence of a TBA or grandmother (known as "gogo"), and my choice of having a home delivery with educated midwives was seen as acceptable. However, I did not plan to tie knots in the umbilical cord to prevent another pregnancy too quickly, or to bury to the placenta and cord as a traditional Swazi woman would do after delivering at her homestead. Complications occurred during my delivery and I was able to get to the hospital quickly for a cesarean section—again unlike many Swazi women, especially those in rural areas.

Throughout my nursing career, since the arrival of my little Leah Lomvula, I have felt the strength of the connection that having a child brings to not only the research process but to professional life as well. When I returned to the United States and took a position with a small college while writing my dissertation, the impact of having a baby remained. My very first day on the job, I had to bring her with me while her father was interviewing for his new job. As I hurried with her into my new office, closing the door quickly behind me, all I could think of was that bringing a baby to work is not professional and certainly not appropriate within our Western culture. I quickly discovered I was wrong: the faculty was eager to hold the new baby and embrace me into the new position as well. My misconceptions about bringing a baby to the workplace—at least for short periods of time—were dispelled and were a source of laughter among the faculty for some months.

My husband, daughter and I returned to Swaziland a few years later as my dream of working with Project HOPE came true. Swazis I had known during my research work again opened their homes and hearts when I arrived with Leah Lomvula, the accelerant of conversation. Weekends were filled with travels to nearby South Africa and throughout Swaziland on safari. One of Leah Lomvula's favorite pastimes was watching the hippos feed on a lazy Sunday afternoon and riding in the back of a worn-out, rusty Range Rover looking for game.

Today, Leah Lomvula is in college, and her love of animals and traveling to foreign lands remains. After Swaziland, she developed a love of horses by living with the Navajo. Leaving the Navajo Nation for Pakistan, we learned about daily life from Pakistani families who welcomed Leah Lomvula and me into their homes. Now, as Leah Lomvula anticipates a return to South Africa this summer for a course on animals in game parks, I can remember where it all began, on a rainy day in Africa.

A Danish Nurse in China

~

Jytte Holst-Bowers, LPN, RN

"THE AMERICAN CONSULATE is looking for a nurse. Why don't you go for it?"

My friend Frances took my arm as we walked across the campus of Zhongshan University in Canton as she asked this question.

"Oh, no, dear friend. I finished with that career long ago."

"Well, I just thought it a good idea. Think it over, won't you?"

I pondered for a couple of days, talking it over with Jim, my husband, who had brought me to Zhongshan University, where he and Frances taught English and where I, together with other spouses, tried the almost impossible task of learning Chinese. At least in the job at the consulate I would be able to speak English, but I didn't remember much from my education as a registered nurse in Denmark over 30 years ago. Yes, I had had some retraining in the United States and worked as a nurse at the college where my husband taught, as well as in nursing homes in Michigan, Colorado, and South Dakota, but a nurse for the U.S. Consulate? That was somewhat doubtful.

Despite my reservations, I did apply for the position. When I learned I'd gotten the job, my pleasure and apprehension were about equal. A couple of days later I hurried through the campus to catch a ferry across the Pearl River to a street in the inner city which was only a few blocks from the consulate in the Dong Fang Hotel. I wasn't the only person on that early morning ferry.

It was early April 1989. A dozen students also walked up the gangplank. They wore white headbands covered with Chinese characters and were searching their pockets for change. Their leader said something to the woman who collected the fares. She shook her head firmly.

"What is this all about?" I turned to a student in the hope that he could speak English.

"Well," he said, "we don't have money. We also pay for lunch. In Beijing, buses let protestors go for free. All students free go to Tiananmen for democracy. Today we also go on march to show friends we care."

"I see," I said, "I'll take care of your fares." I gave the woman the few coins needed. When we reached the other side of the river, the students joined the thousands of young people preparing their peaceful march toward freedom. I walked among the masses of Chinese on the street and reached the consulate just in time for my interview.

My first day at work was not a good beginning. The consulate had invited the doctor, an overseas Chinese woman who was supposed to be my backup, and me to a banquet to celebrate our new association.

"Where is Dr. Ye?" I asked anxiously, sitting at a beautiful lunch table where nothing was missing but the doctor.

"You haven't heard? She is on her way back to America. She has a blood clot in her leg, and they thought it best she be transferred back to the States."

"Oh!" was all I could say as I dropped a delicious Chinese tidbit onto my lap. So there I was, all alone, with no one to guide me.

"But you can always call the American doctor at the embassy in Beijing if you have any questions," he said.

No doubt the doctor was a very capable man, but did the consulate not know how inadequately the Chinese communication system worked in the Year of Our Lord 1989?

Nevertheless, I set up my office and prepared myself for my first patients. The nurse from the embassy in Beijing came visiting, and I received a welcome telegram from the ambassador. I was assured by everyone that I would be fine. No one in the whole world can be more confident than Americans.

"Don't worry," the nurse from Beijing said, "just have your book on nursing procedures standing on a shelf in the bathroom. If you are in doubt, excuse yourself and go to the toilet, research the problem, and find the answer."

Then we went to the market to find a teapot so I could brew myself a cup of tea, like the British nurse at the consulate in Hong Kong, which was close to Canton but not yet a part of the mainland. Over tea, all the world's problems would be solved.

The employees of the consulate were almost all young people who enjoyed a TGIF (Thank God It's Friday) at the end of the week. Their illnesses were of small concern: colds, headaches, diarrhea—much like those of the college students I had nursed ten years earlier. But after the visit of U.S. Surgeon General Dr. C. Everett Koop, the consulate had been anxious to find a hospital sterile enough to meet his demands—in case of an emergency. That was almost impossible to find in China only ten years after the end of the Cultural Revolution. When you visited the wards reserved for party members or foreigners, you might be impressed by how spotless they appeared. The nurses' uniforms were so white and starched they looked like crinolines. But the nurses did not realize that after a needle was inserted intravenously it had to be taped down securely, among other things. As for the hospitals devoted to ordinary Chinese people, they were simply filthy.

The emergency came on June fourth. At 2 a.m. I was called to the phone in the lobby. *Dear God, let it not be the American Consulate telling me the consul has had a heart attack*, I whispered to myself as I left our tiny two-room apartment at Zhongshan University.

It wasn't. It was my husband Jim's mother screaming

into the phone all the way from Connecticut. "You have to come home, I am telling you. You have to come home. They are burning them. The buses are burning. The people are burning. You have to come home!"

The students who had gathered at Tiananmen Square for the last few months had been attacked by the Chinese army. Some of those students were from our university and had traveled to Beijing to show their solidarity with their fellow students. My husband had gathered his graduate students in our apartment when he taught them a course in American literature. One of them had been the leader of the nightly marches out of the front gate of our university and into the city to join the young people from the other colleges in the city. We would never forget the day that young man quoted, quietly but with determination, "Give me liberty or give me death."

Jim and I—indeed most Americans, including the women and children of the consulate—were ordered to leave China within 48 hours. My two months' work for the American Consulate came to a quick end. I folded my white jacket and went to my boss.

"Goodbye and thank you," I said as I shook his hand.

"Yes, but you will be coming back when all this has blown over, won't you?" he asked.

"I doubt it. This has been too much for my husband and me, but thank you once again."

In 2005, however, we did return to China to teach for one semester. I assisted Jim by helping small groups of students practice their spoken English.

"Why did you leave China when you seemed to have liked it so much?" they asked.

"We left because of Tiananmen," I answered.

Their faces were blank. Later, I learned from Jim's Chinese colleague that the Chinese government had rewritten history: the massacre on Tiananmen Square never occurred. No one is allowed to speak about it. The younger generation knows nothing about the students who sacrificed their lives to the Goddess of Liberty. But on this 20th anniversary we are lighting a candle on the evening of June fourth and placing it in our window in their memory, for we have the freedom to express the sorrow we have felt over and over again—to act on behalf of our Chinese friends who do not have that freedom.

The Lucky Ones

~

Tess Deshefy-Longhi, DNSc, RN

THOSE OF US who have done nursing abroad in Third World countries have very similar stories. I always find it amazing how akin they are despite the passage of time. Mine took place in Kisumu, Kenya, from 1969 to 1971.

They were the lucky ones. Flies buzzed mercilessly around their nostrils—these children with the swollen bellies, indifferent eyes, and blond frizz. They had survived the long journey to the "district hospital" for nourishment that would help them live another day. Listless and feeling poorly, they did not complain. Only the infants cried. The older ones—those two years and older—knew it wouldn't bring relief. So they quietly settled into corners along the hospital walls.

Others were not so lucky. One four-year-old had a

permanent tracheotomy tube, and spoke to us through gestures and facial expressions. It was only a matter of time before the frayed ends of gauze keeping the tube in place would give way. We could replace the gauze before it happened, but who would do this—and with what— once he returned to the *shamba,* the small countryside, or farming area where his family lived How long before he succumbed to a raging respiratory infection?

Another child, born with a partially occluded airway, lay in his mother's arms, struggling for air. The only source of oxygen was a seven-foot tank about 100 feet away—permanently chained to the wall behind the nurses' small desk. I was the only one frantically searching for another, more portable source of oxygen. My two students stayed with the mother and child, and everyone let out long, heart-rending wails of grief when the child died. I stood at the door, empty-handed, breathless. Stunned. That night was the first time I cried since arriving in the country.

How long did it take for us outsiders to finally understand that our beliefs and ways and priorities were not necessarily the "right" beliefs, ways, or priorities for our host country nationals?

We retreated to our little house on the hospital compound, my roommate and I, and we shared our stories from the wards and the classrooms. We were fatigued, and in culture shock, and we laughed at the absurdities we witnessed each day to fend off more tears.

How could this be that there were no "code blues"? How could the students learn if they had no library? We planned and we schemed. What would it take to set up a "crash cart"? Where would we get the equipment for it? There was nothing disposable here. If we could create a library, where would we find books that our students could read? Who would check or run these things we made? We would, for starters; but who would do so in our absence? Whom could we trust with them? How would they teach others to keep them going?

Why couldn't they see the importance of such things? Wasn't life as dear here as it was in the United States? Surely it was just a matter of making them understand *the right way* to do things. Surely it would simply be a matter of time. And time simply moved more slowly in this corner of the world. Surely, surely...*we* slowly came to understand.

Our students taught us. A few of the young women we taught had come to "be a nurse." Most were just grateful for a government-paid education beyond grade school. Many were pleased that now they would bring a higher bride price for their father—and with any luck a better suitor for themselves.

They worked hard for their education. They went to classes or worked on the wards every day except Sunday, and they went home only to spend time with their families twice a year.

They were patient as we expounded on good bedside nursing techniques. They smiled gamely as we drew the body's basic systems on the chalkboard, so they could create their own anatomy and physiology "books." We hoped that they would take these resources with them when they graduated and returned to their villages to take charge of the local dispensaries.

At the end of a full day of classes, they would sometimes talk with us about what they believed in. They argued among themselves over what number wife was the best to be. When we told them there was only one wife for every husband in the United States, they said, "Ah, but sisters, you have guns in America. It is very dangerous. Here we do not have guns."

They taught us the rules of the extended family. Each tribe had its own variation of these rules, and there were no orphanages anywhere in the country. Gently they taught us that we were the ones doing things differently, not them. Our ways were strange, not theirs. And they made allowances for us, telling their parents that even though we were "Americans" we were "peace corpse" volunteers, and that was an entirely different being!

We were the lucky ones. We brought home with us a new respect for the fragility of life. We witnessed the resilience of people who faced significant hardships every day, and we grew stronger because of their examples. We understood, finally, that death is truly a part of living and as such it must be addressed—not beaten back at all costs. And we learned all this from people rich in everything but material goods.

Indeed *we* were the lucky ones.

Breath

~

Joan Cantwell, RN, MA, CJEA

I'VE BEEN TOLD that memory can get stuck in tissue or bone. It hides deep within the body, or tucks itself into the unconscious, waiting for permission and the right time to be revealed. In December of 1996, three months into practicing insight meditation and 17 years after working for the American Refugee Committee (ARC) at Camp Khao-I-Dang, Thailand, the memory of her revealed itself to me.

One night, after I had been meditating for about 20 minutes, a woman's voice disturbed the deep calm of my mind by yelling *You didn't save me!*

I remembered my teacher saying that when any disturbing image or sound appears in the mind's eye, gently acknowledge it without judgment, and return focus to the breath. I attempted to bring my attention back to my breath, but the voice forced itself again into my awareness like an angry genie enraged at being held captive so long. She yelled louder. *You didn't save me!* As I shifted my body in an attempt to escape, her voice continued to follow me, repeating, *You didn't save me.* It was inevitable. I took one deep breath, then entered the past without any hope of having a relaxing meditation.

IT WAS 1980. ARC's adult acute-care hospital was the first in a row of several international hospitals at Khao-I-Dang. We, the Americans, had Hospital One. Across from us was the German Red Cross; down the row were the French, the English, and the Japanese. The buildings looked similar, simple bamboo structures lined with sheets of blue plastic that kept out the intense Thai heat and heavy rains during monsoon season. Our hospital was one large, open room with about 100 plywood platform beds. It was always crowded with medical staff, assistants, translators, patients, their families, and visitors. Sometimes the beds were so crowded we had trouble distinguishing the patients from their family members.

I was the youngest member of ARC's medical team, 22 years old, only seven months out of nursing school, and extremely idealistic. I was chosen by ARC because of my intensive care unit experience, combined with my brief exposure to rural healthcare in the Dominican Republic the summer prior to coming to Khao-I-Dang.

ARC's hospital was as far from Northwestern's ICU as I could have imagined. Back in Chicago, I worked in a high-tech world surrounded by professors, residents, medical students, and a team of bright, eager nurses. I was accustomed to medical emergencies, but help was always nearby, and often the biggest decision I ever had to make by myself was choosing which resident I would have to wake up.

Khao-I-Dang was different. How different, I realized my first week in Thailand, when I had to choose which evacuation team I would be on in the event the increasingly agitated Vietnamese troops near the Thai border attacked. At the hospital, supplies and sometimes staff were scarce. The first time I worked night shift alone, the hospital was full, two patients had active meningococcal meningitis, and I didn't have a crash cart. It was just me, an assistant, and a doctor on call from one of the other hospitals who didn't speak much English. I remember getting medical orders that night that had been translated from English to Khmer to French, then back to English again.

One 110-degree afternoon, after I had finished passing meds, Doctor Bob asked me to take a female patient for a chest X-ray to a different part of the camp. He was busy with other patients and didn't have time to take her. I was the only medical staff available, something I wasn't concerned about until I saw her.

I've never remembered her name, but I do remember that she looked like a fragile china doll lying by herself without any friends or family around. I could not tell her age—somewhere between 20 and 60. War has a habit of aging people, distorting the years between birth and death.

Her eyes were dark, sunken ovals focused somewhere far beyond me and time. Her skin, a shiny yellow-green color, hung loosely over thin limbs. Her abdomen was grossly distended and stretched tight with fluid, like an overfilled balloon ready to pop with any additional pressure.

Her diagnosis was Chinese liver fluke disease. According to my Centers for Disease Control manual, this was supposed to be a chronic disease, sometimes with a duration of 30 years or more, and often not a direct or contributing cause of death. Apparently, the liver flukes didn't give a damn about the CDC. Nor did they care that their host had walked 100 land-mined miles from Cambodia to get here, or that on the way she had witnessed her husband gunned down in front of her, or that she had voluntarily drunk infested river water in order to stay alive long enough to make it to the Thai-Cambodian border.

The flukes were only playing out their role as predators, waiting for the right method of entry from the weakest host that came their way. How ironic to survive the trials and violence of a four-year genocide only to face death by drinking the wrong water! How many times back in Chicago had I taken clean water for granted? Mindlessly drinking it, unaware of its powerful ability to save or destroy.

This woman's case was already advanced. She had severe liver damage, extensive abdominal swelling, and now profound shortness of breath. Bob had wanted a chest X-ray to see if fluid had infiltrated her lungs, and if so, he would do a pleural tap to temporarily alleviate her labored breathing. We all understood she was critically ill and that there was not much we could do medically other than to treat each symptom and keep her comfortable. We did not officially chart Do Not Resuscitate in camp as we would have in the States. I assumed we all thought she was DNR, but I didn't realize that I'd soon be the person to have to decide.

The X-ray building was about a quarter mile away, in a different part of the camp. I was concerned about moving my patient. She was using so much energy to breathe that I feared any additional movement might aggravate her condition. Yet we needed an X-ray. A volunteer driver helped me carefully lift her from the bed onto a gurney and into the back of a dusty pickup truck. She glanced briefly at me, then fixed her eyes back into space as we moved her.

I sat next to her in the back of the truck, mopping her brow and shooing the anxious flies away from her eyes. Why did they always swarm around the sickest people? Did they sense when a person's spirit was preparing to leave, or did they have some complex radar system that tuned into death? Damn flies, I hated them. In our hospital they would line up on the pink string we had strung across the room to hang patient IVs on. I think they liked the sticky antibiotics that leaked onto the string. At night, when the camp was asleep and we made rounds, those strings, now black, would hum in unison, as if mocking us—"They're ours, go home." Years later, back in the United States, I'd scrub my skin raw if a fly landed on me.

As the truck pulled away, three small, disheveled girls ranging from ages five to 12 suddenly appeared from somewhere within the camp and filed in line quietly behind the truck, fixing their eyes directly on my patient, their mother. They walked silently, like stoic little soldiers guarding their mother's journey, as if their company were her lifeline, keeping her breathing just a little longer. The Jeep crept slowly through camp. We drove past the refugees' living quarters—140,000 Cambodian, Vietnamese, and Chinese refugees living in a two-by-two-mile perimeter. We drove slowly past tiny bamboo huts that often housed up to three families at a time. Children ran past the truck playing with their bamboo toys; women walked calmly, perhaps on their way to receive their daily rationed water or to socialize at the camp's market, where the scent of freshly made bread lingered in the air. Swarming flies, 110-degree heat, dust-covered bodies, rationed water, no privacy, and the children played on.

Our truck pulled up to the X-ray building and the driver and I carefully moved our patient inside and onto the X-ray table. Her children stood quietly outside and waited for us to return. During the X-ray her breathing became increasing labored, so when the X-ray was completed, we moved quickly to get her back into the truck. I motioned to the driver to hurry up and the children, aware of my increasing anxiety, began crying as they ran after the truck.

I prayed she would not die while we were still in the truck. I tried a couple of Hail Mary's. They always worked for my grandmother when she felt panicked and for me on airplanes, one Hail Mary on takeoff and one on landing. Now, in my panic, I prayed, "Mary, please don't let this woman die now." Not now, not in the middle of this camp, not with me alone to attend to her, and especially not with her children watching.

But Khao-I-Dang was Buddha's territory, and he is a brutal realist. His miracles are performed through insight, not some miraculous recovery. I could hear him correcting me, perhaps even laughing, as he translated my pleas to Mary: *What she really means is, Mary save me from my own fear.* Fear of being alone without my medical team, fear of not knowing what to do, fear of the children's anxiety, but mostly fear of the deep sighs and the labored breathing that I knew came before the final letting go.

As the woman's breathing slowed, my racing mind flooded with questions. *Do I attempt to resuscitate her? Should I assume she was a DNR, and if so, was I right? Is that what the medical team would do? What could I possibly do for her anyway? What good was CPR?*

There was no crash cart, no ambu bags, no medical team to help me decide, nothing familiar from the rooms of Northwestern Memorial Hospital in Chicago. Nothing but the sight of the three small, dirty faces staring up at me from behind the truck, their eyes pleading with me to save their mother, save them from becoming orphans, more casualties of the war they had so far managed to survive.

I did not do CPR and she died, in Khao-I-Dang, on the back of the truck with the impatient flies, the dust, the unending heat, the primitive technology, and the lingering scent of market bread.

Back at the hospital, after seeing how upset I was, Doctor Bob and the rest of the team calmly assured me I had done the "right thing." But I was still plagued with questions. *Had I played God? Made the wrong decision? Even if I had done CPR, how much longer would she have lived? And what about my role to "save" and to respond? Had I failed? Or worse yet—not even tried? Did I for one minute have the power to give breath and refuse it?*

And I wondered if her spirit lingered. Did she hover above the truck to watch her children one last time, wondering about their future now without an adult to help them resettle, as perhaps she gave them one final blessing? Or, without hesitating, did she move swiftly toward the light to welcome the pure freedom of breath without pain?

NOW, YEARS LATER, I sit in my living room. My awareness returns to my breath, which has been stuck somewhere low in my abdomen. And I hear her voice call again, this time softer: *You did not save me.* The tightness in my stomach has moved into my chest. I sense that I have been breathing shallowly for a very long time. And, I hear the Buddha say, *All breath moves toward wholeness.* I adjust my position on the cushion, straighten my spine, and allow breath to flow through my body, releasing the voice of 17 years. I answer, *No, I did not save you. I could not save you.*

I believe that it is not through the "doing" that we become healers, but through our ability to bear witness, to be present, to attend to—like my breath during meditation—the breath that grounds, the breath that heals. I bathe in my breath, I can breathe, and I have breath. And from somewhere deep within my body, the question arises.

How does it feel not to have control? How does it feel to let go?

Acknowledgment
of Permissions

"ICE CREAM DAYS" is excerpted from *The Making of a Nurse* by Tilda Shalof, 2007. Published by McClelland & Stewart Ltd. Used with permission of the publisher.

Reader's Guide

1. In the stories "Carmelita's Hands" and "Mae Mae," two young women's lives are forever changed when deformities that defined the entirety of their young lives are repaired by medical teams from the United States. In what ways might these young women's lives be different now than before their surgeries? Discuss the challenges a person in any culture might have if he or she has a physical difference.

2. Nursing, whether in your home country or one very different from your own, can be stressful. The stories "Avenging Vultures," "In the Doghouse," and "Always Pack White Underwear" underscore the importance of maintaining a sense of humor during stressful times. Do you think this concept might be applied to work anywhere? How does one maintain a sense of humor during difficult times? Besides humor, what are other healthy coping mechanisms to alleviate stress?

3. In "Waterlife," John Fiddler finds an innovative way to get around the cultural norm in Chad that men

must always come first. Discuss his methods of triage and other ways of working within a different culture, respecting the local mores, but still accomplishing the work that must be done.

4. Many contributors speak of the difficulty of not knowing the local language when working abroad; however, others acknowledge that the principles of patience, compassion, and cultural sensitivity speak volumes in any language. Discuss these ideas. Is it necessary to know the language in order to work effectively? Have you ever cared for a patient who spoke a different language? How did you manage? What supports, if any, did your workplace provide?

5. Clean water is essential to good health. Problems with access are most severe in the developing world, where people perish every year from water-related diseases and also suffer without access to water for their basic needs. Several stories address the huge problem of the lack clean water in the third world. Discuss this statement: *Water is a fundamental global health issue.* Defend your position.

6. Many of the stories in *Nurses Beyond Borders* speak of working in a country with limited resources. The authors learned to do what they could with what they had. Discuss the recurrent theme of scarcity in the Third World. In her story "Burst Wide Open,"

Heather McLeod writes, "I want to step out of the denial that living in the United States affords me..." What do you think she means by this? Discuss the ideas of *plenty* and *scarcity*.

7. In "Frog Leaves, Sage, and Cedar," Julia Quiring-Emblen tells of many traditions of the First Nations people of British Columbia and discusses how their healthcare is like, and different from, her own nursing practice. How do you feel about incorporating nontraditional practices into your nursing practice? What are some of the similarities and differences mentioned in this story to Western medical and nursing practice?

8. Many of the stories in *Nurses Beyond Borders* contain the theme of death as a part of life. In the story "The Lucky Ones," Tess Deshefy-Longhi writes, "... death is truly a part of living and as such it must be addressed—not beaten back at all costs." Discuss this notion. In what ways does Western medical and nursing practice address this model? In what ways does it not?

9. In, "A Midwife in Laos," Maribeth Diver states that "every single healthcare provider—especially midwives—holds fast to deep-rooted clinical beliefs and practices. And this is no less true for practitioners in underprivileged countries." Do you agree, or disagree? Discuss the statement and defend your stance.

10. It has been said that nursing involves both art and science. In, "Breath," Joan Cantwell says that "it is not through the 'doing' that we become healers, but through our ability to bear witness, to be present." Discuss the concepts of "being" versus "doing" in relationship to nursing practice. Is one the "art" and the other the "science"? Does one carry more weight than the other, or is it the balance of the two that is most important? Discuss specific examples of "being" and "doing" in the stories of *Nurses Beyond Borders*.

About the Contributors

SUE AVERILL RN, MBA is co-founder of the nonprofit "One Nurse at a Time" (*www.OneNurseAtATime.org*), an organization that helps nurses become involved in volunteer and humanitarian nursing at home and internationally. She works half the year as an emergency room nurse in Seattle, the other half volunteering around the world with Doctors without Borders and other organizations. She is currently writing a book about her missions in Darfur, Uganda, Ethiopia, and South Sudan. Without the loving support of her friends, she says, none of this would have been possible.

JOAN CANTWELL, RN, MA, CJEA, is a nurse, artist, writer, and expressive arts professor. She provides expressive arts services for patients at Horizon Hospice in Chicago; teaches expressive arts at Roosevelt, DePaul, and Dominican Universities; and consults in health and wellness. Joan is founder of Mindful Living Productions, an organization that provides creative arts services within healthcare industries. She lives in River Forest, Iliinois, with her husband, David.

MARY CATLIN, BSN, MPH, is a freelance public health nurse who works in communicable disease control.

CHERIE CLARK, RN, is a courageous, giving woman who embodies a love that transcends color, race, religion, and politics. She is fiercely determined to give all children a chance in life of which fate has seemingly cheated them. Cherie founded the International Mission of Hope and worked to place thousands of children with adoptive parents, and expanded her work in India and Vietnam to caring for the elderly and helping with disaster relief and reforestation through her own Clark Foundation. Cherie's work has included the building of rural healthcare clinics, including one in My Lai. She spends most of her time in India and Vietnam.

J. CLOUD, RMA, was born in Poole, England, and grew up in the United States and Zimbabwe. She graduated from nursing school in 1999. Her nursing specialties are cardiology, dermatology, surgery, trauma surgery, and pediatric burns unit. She has had bush training and worked three years in the field with the nongovernmental organization Make It Happen Africa (*www.MakeItHappenAfrica.com*). J's passion is to fix the children that no one wants, and teach them how to love.

ELIZABETH COULTER, RN, is an emergency room nurse who loves to write. She is currently working on a novel, *Scrubless—The Dysfunctional World of an* ER *Nurse*. She has worked in Canada, England, Hawaii, and Seattle, and volunteered in China with Love Without Boundaries (*www.lovewithoutboundaries.com*) and in Vietnam. She encourages all nurses to volunteer in other countries so their passion for nursing will remain strong.

TESS DESHEFY-LONGHI, DNSC, RN, is a nurse researcher and postdoctoral fellow at the Center for Aging and Human Development, Duke University Medical Center. She was a Peace Corps volunteer in Kisumu, Kenya, where she taught student nurses at the Nyanza Provincial Hospital School of Nursing. She lives in Durham, North Carolina with her husband.

MARIBETH DIVER, CNM, MSN, is a certified-nurse midwife who spent 2001–2003 working in Laos. She now does home, birth center, and hospital deliveries in rural Lancaster County, Pennsylvania, working primarily with Old Order Amish families.

MARTHA N. EZELL, MSN, BSN, was a stay-at-home mom for 15 years, after which she returned to school and became a registered nurse. Her decision was prompted by a medical mission trip to Honduras. She obtained BSN and MSN degrees from Belmont University in Nashville, Tennessee. After working in several nonprofit clinics in Nashville, she found a professional home teaching nursing students at Belmont. Martha and her husband, Mark, have four children. She serves on the advisory boards of

Faith Family Medical Clinic, Hope Clinic for Women and, the Jovenes en Camino orphanage in Honduras.

JOHN B. FIDDLER, RN, ANP, was born in Dublin, Ireland, and has lived in New York City since 1984. Originally pursuing a career in fashion, he was inspired to become a nurse after witnessing the devastation of AIDS in the city. After graduation in 1998 he worked as a critical-care burn nurse, including working with survivors of the 9/11 attacks. After receiving his master's degree in nursing in 2004 from Hunter-Bellevue School of Nursing in New York City, he joined Doctors Without Borders. He currently works as a palliative care nurse practitioner in Queens, New York.

ANNA GERSMAN, RN, BSCN, grew up in a large family near Toronto, Canada. She has practiced nursing in South Africa and the Caribbean, and for the last 12 years has worked as a home-care case manager. She lives near Toronto with her husband of 25 years and their teenage daughters, Ariel and Liora.

GRACE HATMAKER, RN, MSN, PHD STUDENT, has a master's in nursing from Widener University and a bachelor's in nursing from Villanova University. She is a full-time doctoral student with the University of Nebraska Medical Center, focusing on childhood injury prevention in the Hmong refugee population. She also teaches a master's seminar for clinical nurse specialists at California State

University, Fresno. Grace's clinical background has always been related to emergency nursing and pediatrics with a clinical nurse specialty in burn/emergency/trauma.

JYTTE HOLST-BOWERS, LPN, RN, was born in Copenhagen, Denmark, in 1931 and trained as a registered nurse at Bispebjerg Hospital. In 1959 she married James Bowers from Connecticut. They have four children: three married daughters and a son with Down syndrome. She has written a memoir about their life together, including teaching in Finland, China, Czechoslovakia, and Lithuania. Her husband and she enjoy their retirement in a log cabin in the Black Hills of South Dakota, reading, writing, and living a simple life.

SARAH LIBERMAN, RN, MSN is a passionate registered nurse who enjoys finding creative ways to contribute to the profession. Her clinical background with vulnerable populations both at home and abroad grounds her work endeavors in the experiences of clients. She holds a master's of nursing from the University of Saskatchewan. Her research interests include advocacy, social justice, critical social theory, health equity, global health, and qualitative and community-based methods. Sarah currently works in health policy addressing health disparities. She has an insatiable appetite for learning, traveling, and chocolate.

FIONA MACLEOD, BSN, is a Canadian nurse who completed her bachelor's in nursing at Trent University,

Peterborough, Ontario. Since graduating in 2004, she has worked in both clinical and research settings including rural health in Honduras; HIV and addictions in Vancouver, British Columbia; and currently, oncology in Riyadh, Saudi Arabia. In the future, Fiona hopes to pursue her passion for cross-cultural care, which she feels brings deeper meaning both to her practice and her personal fulfillment.

HEATHER STARSHINE MCLEOD, MSN, ARNP, is an advanced registered nurse practitioner living in Washington State. She currently specializes in Women's Health and Family Planning, and also works as a sexual-assault nurse examiner. She has volunteered in Africa, Latin America, and Asia, and loves the opportunity for the eye-opening adventures that being a nurse provides.

JOYCE MUELLER, RN, says that retired life on the Oregon coast has given her the time to write her story about learning to be a *memsahib* in East Pakistan in the 1960s. Her next book will be about her life in West Pakistan, followed by tales from four years in the Solomon Islands. She states that she's never going to have to die. Widowed, Joyce has three loving sons and families and outstanding supportive friends. She can be reached at 541-332-0133.

PAULA NANGLE, RN, BA, MFA, lives in Michigan, where she is employed as a psychiatric nurse. Her work has appeared in *Glimmer Train*, *Michigan Quarterly Review*,

Crab Orchard Review, and other publications, and is forth-coming in *HOW Journal*. Her novel, *The Leper Compound*, was published by Bellevue Literary Press in 2008.

CONNIE NUNN, RN, BN, has been a nurse for 35 years. She started her career in international health as a volun-teer nurse with the Canadian organization CUSO in Sierra Leone in 1980. Since her first mission, Connie has helped implement healthcare activities in countries throughout Africa and Asia, including Tajikistan, Sudan, Pakistan, and Ghana. For the past ten years she has worked with International Medical Corps, and she has served the past four years as a site manager for the organization's pro-gram in Darfur, Sudan.

JULIA QUIRING-EMBLEN, PHD, RN, received her BSN from the University of Oregon, and MSN and PhD from the University of Washington. She has taught medical-surgical and community health nursing. Her most recent focus has been on spiritual care. After retiring from Trinity Western University in British Columbia, she worked at Portland Community College and served as consultant for Oregon Coast Community College. Currently she is serving as a parish nurse and developing materials to be used by congregational members to assist them in visiting the homebound.

LOUISE M. ROBINSON, RN, earned her nursing degree at the age of 45, then joined the Peace Corps and was sent to

Guatemala, where she single-handedly enriched the lives of an entire country. Certified as an International Red Cross volunteer nurse, she was sent to Kuwait to assist at a refugee camp. Louise continues to do volunteer work while working as a registered nurse in Colorado. Raising her grandchildren has been only one of her many adventures.

TILDA SHALOF, RN, BSCN, CNCC(C), is a staff nurse in the Medical-Surgical Intensive Care center at Toronto General Hospital and has worked in hospitals in Israel and the United States. She is the author of the best-seller *A Nurse's Story,* which has been translated into numerous foreign languages, as well as *The Making of a Nurse,* and *Camp Nurse;* and is the editor of *Lives in the Balance: Nurses' Stories of the ICU,* in the Nurses' Voices series by Kaplan Publishing. Tilda is an inspiring public speaker, a media commentator, an outspoken patient advocate, and a passionate nursing leader. She lives with her husband, Ivan Lewis, and their two sons in Toronto, Canada, and can be reached at (*www.NurseTilda.com*).

MICHELE J. UPVALL, PHD, RN, FNP, is a professor of nursing at Carlow University in Pittsburgh, Pennsylvania, where she teaches in the master's and doctor of nursing practice programs. She has extensive transcultural and global health experience, including teaching and development and administration of nursing programs in Swaziland, the Navajo Nation, Zanzibar, Pakistan, and Cambodia. Her current research interests are related to

patient advocacy and role development of community health nursing in underdeveloped countries.

JANET M. VOGT, RNFA, BSN, CNOR, has been an operating room nurse for 30 years, the last 16 as pediatric urology co-coordinator at Saint Louis Children's Hospital. She participated in pediatric urology mission trips for over 12 years with International Volunteers in Urology, traveling to Vietnam, India, Mongolia, Cuba, and Ghana. She lives in St. Louis, Missouri, with her husband, their four children, and one daughter-in-law, ranging in ages from 20 to 28.

About the Editor

NANCY LEIGH HARLESS is an award-winning poet, writer, and women's healthcare nurse practitioner. Her stories have been included in many anthologies, including *Kaplan Voices: Nurses, Cup of Comfort, The Healing Project, Chicken Soup for the Soul,* and *Travelers' Tales,* as well as many professional and literary journals. Nancy authored her own collection of short stories gleaned from her international nursing experiences and travel, *Womankind: Connection & Wisdom Around the World,* and served as co-editor for Kaplan Publishing's *To the Rescue: Stories from Healthcare Workers at the Scenes of Disaster.* Nancy travels often—usually off the well-paved road. She completed *Nurses Beyond Borders* while living in San Miguel de Allende, Mexico. Nancy may be reached through her website: *www.womankindconnection.com.*